Leon Chaitow is a leading practitioner of osteopathy, naturopathy and acupuncture. He teaches widely in the United Kingdom, Europe, Australia and the United States of America, and is a senior lecturer at the University of Westminster, London. He practices at the Hale Clinic, London and is the bestselling author of a wide range of health guides.

Thorsons Natural Health

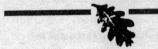

High Blood Pressure

LEON CHAITOW

Thorsons
An Imprint of HarperCollins*Publishers*

Thorsons
An Imprint of HarperCollins*Publishers*
77–85 Fulham Palace Road,
Hammersmith, London W6 8JB

First published by Thorsons 1986
This revised edition 1998
20 19 18 17 16 15 14

A catalogue record for this book
is available from the British Library

ISBN-13 978-0-7225-3563-9
ISBN-10 0-7225-3563-5

Printed and bound in Great Britain by
Clays Ltd, St Ives plc

Contents

Contents

For Sasha

Note to Reader

While the author of this work has made every effort to ensure that the information contained in this book is as accurate and up to date as possible at the time of publication, medical and pharmaceutical knowledge is constantly changing and the application of it to particular circumstances depends on many factors. Therefore it is recommended that readers always consult a qualified medical specialist for individual advice. This book should not be used as an alternative to seeking specialist medical advice, which should be sought before any action is taken. The author and publishers cannot be held responsible for any errors and omissions that may be found in the text, or any actions that may be taken by a reader as a result of any reliance on the information contained in the text, which is taken entirely at the reader's own risk.

Introduction
What is Blood Pressure?

The aim of this book is for you to come to a general understanding of your body, and your blood pressure in particular, as it relates to your health and your life. In so doing you will achieve insights into the marvellous manner in which the body functions and how it is possible for problems to arise in the cardio-vascular system which are directly related to factors over which you have a good degree of control. Hypertension, or as it is commonly called high blood pressure, is one indication of problems arising. It is not a disease as such but a condition which can be life-endangering, and is in fact the leading contributory cause of death in the industrialized countries of the West.

We will look at the dynamics of the cardio-vascular system, and just how blood pressure relates to health; we will investigate the major factors in our lifestyles and diets that can influence it, and above all we will delve into the ways in which problems can be avoided and overcome in this regard.

There is growing realization, in the medical world, that it is necessary for there to be a change in attitude towards disease, away from the idea that there is a 'cure' for everything, via drugs or treatment, and towards the concept of individuals taking personal responsibility for the maintenance and regaining of health. Nowhere is this more true than in the area of hypertension, where simple alterations in diet, exercise and behaviour can often dramatically change a situation in which there is real danger, to one in which healthy function is restored.

If you want to understand what blood pressure is all about, what high blood pressure results from, and its implications; and what you, yourself, can do to avoid or reverse such a problem, then this book is designed for you.

It is not suggested that medical treatment of hypertension is always unnecessary, but it is suggested that drug treatment is frequently used when self-help methods would provide a better and safer long-term solution.

The Circulatory System

Picture the following sequence of events, which takes place within the closed circuit of the circulatory system of the body. The muscular pump, the heart, receives

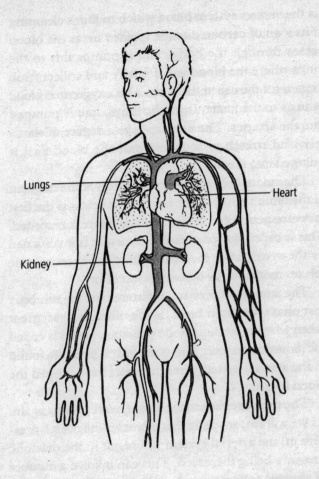

Lungs

Heart

Kidney

Figure 1: The circulatory system

via the venous system blood which requires cleansing of its load of carbon dioxide (picked up as the blood passes through the body) and it pumps this to the lungs where the blood will detoxify and collect fresh oxygen for the use of the body. This oxygenated blood returns to the heart, from the lungs, and is pumped into the arteries. The arteries have a degree of elasticity, and stretch to accommodate the blood as it is pumped into them.

The amount of pressure in the artery at the moment of maximum effort of the heart (as it beats) is the first measurement taken when blood pressure is recorded. This is called *systolic* pressure. Pressure is maintained by the artery after the beat, whilst the heart muscle relaxes momentarily before its next effort.

The amount of pressure registered during this brief rest phase, between beats, is the other measurement taken when recording blood pressure, and it is called the *diastolic* pressure. This is the lowest pressure found in the arterial system after the heart has pumped the blood into it.

The pressure rises again as the heart pumps again. As we will see, anything that increases the overall pressure on the arterial system will result in the diastolic pressure being increased. This can involve a number of possible factors, including the loss of elasticity in the blood vessel walls through hardening, or increased muscular pressure resulting from stressed or tensed muscles pressing on them. Such increased pressure in the blood vessels results in the heart having to pump harder in order to force the blood through them, and the end result of this could reflect in the systolic pressure reading as well.

To summarize what has been said above: the forceful movement of blood being pumped into the arterial system is the systolic pressure, and the rest phase, between beats, when the actual inter-arterial pressure is recorded, is the diastolic pressure.

Taking Blood Pressure

These pressures are measured by an instrument called a sphygmomanometer. Using an air-filled cuff it occludes, or cuts off, the circulation momentarily whilst the sound of the pulse is listened for by means of either a stethoscope or an electronic device. As the heart pumps, the air in the cuff is slowly released until the pressure of the heart matches the pressure of the cuff of the sphygmomanometer. The sound of the pulse heard at that moment signals the systolic level, on a column of mercury. As the heart effort eases, during the rest between beats, the level of mercury drops in its column, and the next 'sound' listened for is that of the cessation of the sound of the pulsation of blood through the artery as the cuff releases its pressure on it. This is the actual pressure level in the artery, also

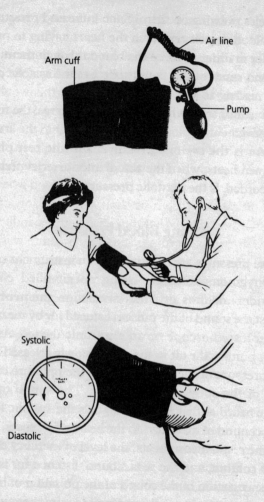

Figure 2: Testing blood-pressure

expressed by the height of the column of mercury, supported by the pressure.

The readings thus taken are recorded, and these are written, or stated, as the systolic figure 'over' the diastolic figure. In the average individual this would be around 120 over 80 (120/80) millimetres of mercury (mm/Hg).

From these two figures much can be deduced about the health of the individual. It should be noted that these figures represent the pressure of blood when the measurement is taken at the usual position of the upper arm, at the level of the heart, with the individual seated and the arm supported. The pressure will vary in different positions (lying down, standing) and in different locations (upper or lower leg, etc.).

It is possible for great variations to exist in pressures under varying conditions and in different positions, and for important diagnostic information to be gathered in this way. However, it is the commonly taken arm pressure that we are referring to, in this instance, as being 'normal' at 120/80/mm/Hg.

It is also worth noting that apprehension or slight tension on the part of the person having his or her pressure taken can alter the accuracy of the reading quite markedly. Thus it has been suggested that the pressure should be taken at least twice, and preferably three times over a 15-minute period, and the last one of all taken as being the most accurate, if the 'anxiety' factor is to be avoided. It was noted, in an Italian trial, that hospital patients about to have their pressure recorded showed an increase in diastolic pressure which was maintained for 10 minutes or more. Thus the practice was introduced of taking the pressure several times, and leaving the sphygmomanometer cuff in position all the while, to overcome the anxiety felt about the procedure.

How Blood Circulation Works

The pumping of the heart (over 100,000 contractions daily) starts the blood on its journey which takes it through a maze of over 60,000 miles of networked vessels. All those carrying fresh, oxygen-rich blood are directed away from the heart, and all those returning 'used' blood for reprocessing (the veins and venules) run towards the heart. The veins, which frequently have to carry blood against the force of gravity, have one-way valves to prevent blood from becoming stagnant, or actually passing the wrong way. It is certainly not possible for the heart action to have the power to pump all the blood all the way around this vast network of tubes, and it is important that we realize that muscular activity, and the action of breathing, have a vital role to play in the whole process of circulation, for these factors are keys to assisting in blood pressure problems.

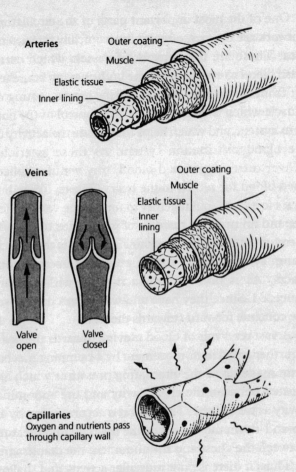

Figure 3: The structure of the blood vessels

One of the most important parts of the circulatory network are the tiny, often microscopically fine arterioles. These are the network of vessels which carry fresh blood to every part of the body, having branched off from the arteries proper. These have a coating of muscle which is directly under the control of the nervous system, and which helps to regulate the activity of the blood distribution system. As these arterioles deliver their oxygenated blood, tiny venules collect used blood for return to the heart. These, like tributaries to a river, join together to form large veins which depend on two vast systems of pumps for the movement of the blood they contain. The first is the muscle pump system. Every time a muscle is used, it contracts. As it does so, veins that lie within it are squeezed. Since they have one-way valves this moves the contents forward (towards the heart).

A vast reservoir of blood moving towards the heart is further aided in its movement by a pumping mechanism made up of the alternating pressures which are created between the chest cavity and the abdominal cavity as we breathe. This action is accompanied by an up-and-down movement of the main dividing feature between the chest and the abdomen: the diaphragm.

Thus, if there is poor muscular activity and shallow breathing, there is likely to be a degree of 'pooling' in the venous system. This can result in a degree of back-pressure building up, affecting the arterial system and thus creating a need for higher pressure from the heart as it beats, or from the muscular coating of the arterial system. This increases the internal pressure of the arteries, and possibly of the heart itself.

Thus on a purely mechanical level it is possible for the blood pressure to be increased through lack of use of the body, and inadequate breathing. Conversely, exercise and proper breathing aid high blood pressure. We will look more closely at exercise and breathing later in the book.

Low Blood Pressure

Blood pressure is vital to life. High blood pressure is a threat to it. There is of course a condition called low blood pressure as well, and we should be aware of its implications. Low blood pressure, or hypotension, is said to exist if an adult has a systolic pressure which is persistently below between 90 and 100mm/Hg. It is usually accompanied by a pulse rate which is rapid but weak, and which will alter, by a reduction of as much as 40 beats per minute, when the individual lies down. There may be no obvious symptoms, but more usually there is a feeling of lassitude, giddiness (especially when standing from the sitting position) and a muzzy head. Fainting may occur at such times. This may in fact be an inherited constitutional state, or it may be the result of any of a number of pathological processes, such as some forms of heart disease, kidney problems, malnutrition, tuberculosis, haemorrhage or physical and mental exhaustion.

The treatment depends upon the cause, of course, but obvious irritants such as the use of purgatives, very hot baths, and excessive prolonged standing should be avoided. The condition is helped by general exercise, and abdominal exercise or support.

As will become clear, the passage of blood returning to the heart can be severely compromised by a number of conditions involving the abdominal area – for example, pregnancy or constipation can send the pressure up, and weak muscular support can cause it to drop. Thus, in low blood pressure from whatever cause the abdominal musculature and breathing mechanism can be used to great effect in assisting the return of blood to the heart. Awareness of low blood pressure as a possible factor in conditions in which there is a feeling of weakness, exhaustion and light-headedness can be useful in pointing to such simple methods of correction.

Breathing function and abdominal tone are of importance in high blood pressure as well, as we will see in the chapters dealing with practical self-help methods of coping with hypertension.

Before continuing to look at the implications of high blood pressure, and a variety of causes for this – most of which lie within the control of the individual to alter

– it will be as well to look briefly at a few of the other factors which can alter the pressure as the blood passes round the body. Anything which causes the blood vessels, through which the blood is passing, to be constricted or narrowed will result in greater pressure being called for to push the blood through them. Thus a variety of factors which can cause increased tension or hardening of the muscular coating of the arteries and arterioles can be responsible, especially if this is a long-term situation. Stress and tension are therefore seen as possible factors in raising pressure. If the arteries and arterioles become narrowed because of deposits within them, then the same thing happens (arteriosclerosis or hardening of the arteries). Since the blood, returning to the heart, has to pass through the kidneys for filtering, the health of these vital organs can influence the pressure. The blood also has to pass through the liver for detoxification and to collect vital nutrients, and so a similar problem can arise if there is less than a healthy liver to work with. Both the liver and the kidneys will be considered in more detail later.

It has been noted that many people have high blood pressure associated with the use of salt, which can alter the biochemical balance in the bloodstream and the body as a whole. Sodium chloride (salt) can produce major imbalances in the biochemical constituency of the body fluids in general, which can increase the degree of effort required by the heart to pump blood, thus raising pressure. As mentioned previously, anything which allows the venous blood to become sluggish in its return to the heart results in back-pressure on the arterial system, also raising the pressure. Such factors as chronic constipation, abdominal tumours, pregnancy, poor muscular tone in the limbs and abdomen, combined with inadequate exercise, can all be contributors to such a state of affairs. Smoking can be a key factor in raising pressure by virtue of its action in constricting the small blood vessels. The use of certain drugs (such as the Pill) can have a similar effect in sensitive individuals.

It is worth noting, of course, that we are all biologically and biochemically individual. Thus factors which affect one person may not affect another at all, or to the same degree. There are many people eating lashings of salt, and smoking heavily, with relatively normal blood pressure (at least for the time being).

If we are to deal satisfactorily with an individual's hypertension problems, then all major factors must be looked at and those implicated as being possible causes should be dealt with, mainly by self-help methods. In this way the marvellous self-repairing mechanisms of the body can begin to restore normal function.

One of the most important causes of increased blood pressure, which is frequently within our control, is overweight. For every pound of excess weight that is carried, there are a hundred miles of extra capillaries (tiny blood vessels) for the heart to push blood through. The effect of being just a little overweight can therefore be a key factor in the blood pressure picture.

Some possible causes of high blood pressure, as outlined above, will be more closely examined in the chapters that follow. First, however, we must look at the implications of high blood pressure to see just what it can mean in terms of life and health.

1
The Implications of High Blood Pressure

High blood pressure can be shown to reduce severely the life expectancy of the individual. A rise to a level of only 130/90mm/Hg, which until recently was thought to be so small a rise as to be unworthy of attention, is shown to cut male life expectancy (at age 35) by four years. A rise at that age to a level of 140/95mm/Hg knocks an estimated (by the Society of Actuaries) nine years off life expectancy.

By the time blood pressure has reached a level of 150/100mm/Hg at age 35, a not uncommon level in modern life, the reduction in anticipated life is over 16 years. Not only this, but the quality of that life can be severely disrupted and lowered, because of the increased risk of becoming an invalid for many of those remaining years due to coronary heart disease, stroke or congestive heart failure.

In long-term studies conducted in the US it was shown that the risks of one or other of these disasters occurring is often trebled when blood pressure rises above normal. In the case of congestive heart failure, the risk is quadrupled.

Every possible factor in causing such a rise is therefore of the greatest importance since, as will be seen, many of the causes are capable of being eliminated from the scene, and the condition can thus frequently be restored to a close approximation of normality.

Since there is no single, clear-cut cause of high blood pressure, there can be no standardized form of therapy. The total combined history of stresses, inherited factors, dietary indiscretions and lifestyle all combine to interact with the particular physiology and psychology of the individual, creating a situation in which the body may have to attempt to maintain circulatory function by means of raising the blood pressure. A drug prescribed to counteract this would either aim at fluid elimination by increasing the kidney output (i.e. a diuretic drug) or it might attempt to expand the contracted blood vessel (i.e. a vasodilatory drug), thus reducing the effort of the heart in pumping the blood through the vessels.

These are symptom-orientated methods. They see the high blood pressure as the entity that requires altering. The drug may well succeed in altering the situation, by lowering the pressure. This, though, would not necessarily be either desirable or scientifically acceptable, since all that would have been achieved would be to have left the underlying causes unchanged. The issue is not whether blood pressure can be speedily lowered by drug methods, for often it can, but whether this is the correct way of approaching a complex problem.

If there is fluid retention, is it not more appropriate to remove the reasons for this? A natural, non-drug programme will do this in many cases, and will bring with it all sorts of additional health bonuses. The drug approach not only does nothing for the underlying causes, but brings with it inevitable side-effects, some of which are potentially very dangerous.

What Affects Blood Pressure?

Blood pressure is the force exerted by the blood within the arteries. It depends upon a number of interacting variables, such as the force of the heart beat, the elasticity of the blood vessel walls; the resistance, or back-pressure, from the body as a whole (such factors as fluid levels and weight influence this); as well as the degree of muscular pressure on the small blood vessels; the viscosity (thickness) of the blood, and its total volume. All these factors have an effect upon the pressure, as do the relative health and efficiency of the liver and kidneys, and the tone and efficiency of the muscular and respiratory (breathing) systems of the body. There are many ways in which a combination of these factors can create a situation which calls for the body to raise the pressure abnormally, and we can frequently normalize the situation by our own efforts by removing causative factors.

There are also many situations in which blood pressure may rise, and yet not be significant or be a cause for concern. It is not uncommon, for example, for the more easily influenced aspect of the blood pressure (systolic blood pressure) to be raised, under upsetting or stressful conditions. This is not considered of any great importance, as long as the other part of the blood pressure remains relatively normal (the diastolic pressure). In some people there is a tendency for the pressure to rise quite rapidly, but it settles towards normal just as fast. This is of interest, but not of great significance. The critical influence which high blood pressure can have on the health of the individual is now much more clearly understood.

It used to be thought that blood pressure necessarily rose with age. In fact it was commonly held that the systolic pressure ought to be somewhere around a figure of 100 plus the age of the individual. This is now known to be totally inaccurate, since blood pressure ought not vary greatly with age, and when it does, it is no more than evidence of the effects of those aspects of life which mitigate against the pressure reading remaining at a normal level.

In societies in which diet has remained relatively unaffected by modern trends, and in which an unpolluted and peaceful existence has been maintained, blood pressure remains at youthful levels into old age, and coronary disease is almost unknown. The blood pressure level enjoyed in early adult life, if health is normal, is the level which is ideal throughout life. The average desirable levels are thought to be in the region of 120 systolic and 80 diastolic, and anything in excess of this is thought to be undesirable. Dangerous implications are considered possible if the pressure is over 160 systolic or 96 diastolic. Levels between the desired 120/80 and the dangerous 160/95 are of importance as they indicate that there is a trend away from normal towards danger, and that action is called for.

Hypertension

Hypertension is the leading physiological abnormality contributing towards death in Western society. In the UK it is the major contributory factor in heart disease and strokes, which together comprise by far the major causes of death. The sad fact is that most people suffering from high blood pressure do not know it, and the longer the condition remains undiagnosed, the greater the chances of it causing damage. It is the lack of symptoms of an obvious nature which frequently prevents many people from being aware of their condition of high blood pressure. It can, and often does, produce symptoms (see below), but more often than not these are absent or so mild as to be taken as part of normal existence. In some people blood pressure fluctuates dramatically depending upon such underlying factors as stress or food sensitivities. In most, though, the pressure just gradually creeps upwards, unnoticed.

Some or all of the following symptoms may accompany hypertension:

Ringing or buzzing in the ears, or a loudly audible
    pulsing in the head.
Frequent nosebleeds.
Dizziness, especially when altering position (although
    low blood pressure may also be responsible).
Headaches or a feeling of fullness in the head.
Alterations in the heart rate, including palpitations.
Frequency of urination.
Swollen lower limbs.
Unexplained irritability.
Unexplained aches and pains.
Unnatural tiredness.

It is just as likely, however, that none of the above will be noticed and that blood pressure will be high without symptoms.

There are also, it should be noted, many people who are born with a natural tendency towards a higher blood pressure than average. Family tendencies towards this are not uncommon and call for special attention to the problem.

The commonly held view that sodium, derived from salt, is a key to high blood pressure is now known to be only part of the picture, and we will consider this in greater detail in a later chapter. What has emerged is that far from salt automatically sending blood pressure up, it is the case that this happens only in those people born with a predisposition to high blood pressure, who are also what is known as 'salt sensitive'. When such individuals are exposed to an average salt intake, they show signs of higher blood pressure. Other individuals can apparently ingest larger amounts of salt without this effect. This illustrates the genetic or inborn nature of hypertension in many people, and shows that simplistic solutions, such as everyone cutting down on salt, would be likely to achieve only partial success because a limited section of the public is salt sensitive with a predisposition towards high blood pressure.

Once high blood pressure is a fact, the amount of damage that can result will also vary considerably from person to person. Many other factors, some inborn, some acquired, will decide just who will succumb to coronary disease or stroke, or who will indeed survive to old age in apparent good health despite hypertension. This is not in any way meant to suggest that hypertension should be ignored, only that its effect will not be uniformly harmful. In the main it is safe to say that health will be better if pressure is low or normal, rather than if it is high. Statistically, life expectancy is greater, and levels of well-being into old age are better if pressure is normal.

It is important for blood pressure to be monitored at regular intervals, especially if there is any family history of cardiovascular disease or of high blood pressure. This can be done by regular visits to a health professional, or by the use of simple self-monitoring equipment which is now available at relatively low cost.

Since high blood pressure is a potential risk to life itself, and since it is also, as we will see, relatively easy in most cases to control by self-help methods, there is every reason for paying attention to this vital health indicator. This does not mean becoming obsessed with health matters, but that, at regular intervals, say once every six months, blood pressure should be checked.

It is a legitimate question to ask whether there is any need for self-help, since there are a variety of drugs available which can control hypertension. There is no doubt that under certain conditions anti-hypertensive drugs are called for, especially in short-term use, if the pressure is dangerously high. However, there is abundant evidence that all such drugs have side-effects (see next chapter), some very serious, and that blood pressure is controllable by safe non-drug methods in the majority of cases. Such non-drug methods may well also bring many other health benefits with them, as well as being infinitely satisfying by virtue of the knowledge that the condition has been dealt with personally, and that causes have been tackled, rather than symptoms alone.

Many esteemed medical authorities have come to the view that drug therapy for hypertension is at best of short-term value, and that the type of measures that will be presented in subsequent chapters offer a far more scientific and acceptable alternative. This is because of growing evidence that drug control of hypertension, whilst apparently effective in achieving symptomatic control, has little overall benefit in terms of increasing life-expectancy or in preventing ultimate cardio-vascular disease from emerging. In contrast, lifestyle and dietary alterations, together with behavioural reforms which combine to lower high blood pressure, confer distinct benefits to the individual in regard to life-expectancy, as well as enhancing overall health. This then is not so much a way of avoiding drugs for no good reason, but of a better, safer and more efficient way of dealing with a major health problem.

If you wish to avoid cardiovascular disease, heart attacks, thrombosis, strokes, angina and myriad other possible complications of hypertension, then the advice contained in the chapters that follow should be studied, understood and applied.

Areas of importance to which we must apply ourselves are those which explain just how different factors can produce high blood pressure. After that we will be ready to look at methods of avoiding these occurrences and of dealing with existing hypertension.

2
More About Blood Pressure

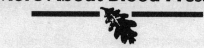

There are a number of important clues that we can obtain from blood pressure readings which can tell us much about the general function of the body and its health status.

As explained in the Introduction, when blood pressure is taken by use of a sphygmomanometer a cuff compresses the artery carrying blood down the arm and it imparts two figures: the systolic pressure measures (in millimetres of mercury, written mm/Hg) the actual pressure required to stop the circulation, the pressure inside the artery itself; the diastolic pressure is the pressure exerted by the heart as it pumps the blood. The two figures are recorded as the systolic pressure 'over' the diastolic pressure – say 120/80 – which would be a normal reading.

If the diastolic blood pressure (the lower of the two figures) is consistently higher than 95 there exists the possibility of problems relating to either the liver (the body's main organ of detoxification) or the kidneys, and further investigation may be called for.

How Hard Is the Heart Working?

There is more information to be gathered than these two figures, however, for example if we wish to establish what is known as the 'workload' of the heart we can do a simple calculation in which we multiply the pulse rate (number of beats of the heart per minute) by the systolic blood pressure (the higher of the two figures taken). The normal figure resulting from such a sum would range between 8,000 and 9,500. Should it amount to something in excess of 9,500, then there is a chance of problems arising in either the kidneys or the liver, or there may be atherosclerotic developments (fatty deposits building up on the inside of blood vessels and restricting blood flow), and further investigation is called for. If, however, the total arrived at is below 8,000, then there is a chance of either what is called 'adrenal insufficiency' (in which the hormonal production of the adrenal glands is below normal for some reason) or there may be a degree of nutritional deficiency or generalized weakness. These would also require investigation and could possibly be dealt with nutritionally. So the 'workload' represents just how hard the heart has to work, being the product of the number of times it beats multiplied by the force with which it beats.

Adrenal Insufficiency

It is possible to obtain additional information from the blood pressure reading about the status of the adrenal glands (which produce that most important hormone, adrenaline). This involves having the blood pressure taken when lying down (after being in that position for at least four minutes) and then immediately after standing up. There should be a rise in the systolic pressure of at least 5 mm/Hg on standing. If not, then the adrenal glands are considered to be weak, under strain or depleted, and action is called for to restore them to normal. This might involve stress-reduction, adequate exercise and rest, and nutritional support as outlined in later chapters, as well as the avoidance of stimulants such as drugs, caffeine, alcohol and cigarettes, which put stress on the adrenal glands.

Testing for High Blood Pressure

There are simple home tests which can be carried out to assess whether there is a potential for the development of high blood pressure as a result of back-pressure on the venous system. This back-pressure can also be taken, to some extent, as an indication of the current efficiency of liver function, at least as far as any influence liver function has on the circulating blood.

With the balls of the thumbs, press down on a fleshy part of the legs (or chest or between the shoulder blades, if you are testing someone else) for about five seconds. The pressure should not be heavy but of medium intensity (enough to cause discomfort but not pain if you were using that amount of pressure on the closed eyes). Release the pressure – if a blanched, white area remains visible, it indicates that increased vein pressure exists. Normal vein pressure would not allow a white area to remain.

Such venous back-pressure can result from a sequence of events which can include either the liver or the kidneys being unable to handle adequately the filtering of blood that passes through them. This can eventually result in extra effort being required from the heart muscle which pumps blood. Back-pressure can also impair circulation to, and through, these vital organs themselves, leading to stress on them and possible future problems.

The elevation of blood pressure via this type of sequence is therefore a secondary event, following on from original problems in the major organs involved. Evidence of such back-pressure in someone with no evidence of high blood pressure can be taken as an indication of problems as yet in their early stages. Attention to the basic requirements of the body, in terms of diet, exercise and stress-reduction, will go a long way to minimizing the likelihood of further degenerative or pathological changes.

In medical terminology the following are the actual definitions of different levels of blood pressure:

- If the **diastolic** pressure reading is 85 mm/Hg or lower, then it is classified as 'Normal'.
- Between 85 and 89 mm/Hg is classified as 'High Normal Blood Pressure'.
- Between 90 and 104 mm/Hg is classified as 'Mild Hypertension'.
- From 105 to 114 mm/Hg is classified as 'Moderate Hypertension'.
- Above 115 mm/Hg is classified as 'Severe Hypertension'.
- The **systolic** reading is regarded as 'Normal' if it is less than 140 mm/Hg (assuming the diastolic pressure to be normal).
- Between 140 and 159 mm/Hg is classified as 'Borderline Isolated Systolic Hypertension'.
- Above 160 mm/Hg is classified as 'Isolated Systolic Hypertension'.
- When the pressure is between 90 and 104 mm/Hg diastolic, and/or 140 and 199 mm/Hg systolic, there is a need to re-check the pressure at least every two months.

- If diastolic pressure exceeds 105 mm/Hg and/or the systolic exceeds 200 mm/Hg, then detailed and speedy evaluation of the condition is called for by a medical or naturopathic practitioner.

In general, then, if the combined blood pressure reading is anything above 140/90, it is above normal.

This degree of abnormality, potential hypertension, applies to around half the adult population of industrialized societies.

Because even this relatively small increase from normal carries a greater risk of cardio-vascular disease and early death, it is important to have blood pressure monitored regularly, especially as there exist a number of safe and effective methods for reducing hypertension naturally, without drugs, in most instances.

In some cases, however, anti-hypertensive drugs – among the most widely prescribed of all medication – are called for, even though long-term tests show that in many instances, while reducing blood pressure, they have little effect on long-term survival potential.

In fact, some recent studies which involved many hundreds of people with high blood pressure over a long period of time suggest that doing nothing at all about high blood pressure is often a better option in survival terms than using anti-hypertension medication.

A far better option than doing nothing, however, is to deal with the (usually) obvious causes of high blood pressure by employing methods which deal with these rather than largely ignoring causes and simply attacking the symptom by pushing the pressure downwards by means of drugs. Such methods – for examining and altering the causes of high blood pressure – will be outlined later in this book.

Later in this chapter there will also be an examination of some of the most common medical treatments for hypertension.

Caution

The self-help advice contained in this book can successfully be applied to the prevention of hypertension, as well as to the treatment of any stage of hypertension. However, should the diastolic pressure exceed 105 mm/Hg and/or the systolic exceed 200 mm/Hg, then the methods outlined should be combined with advice and/or treatment from a qualified health care professional.

Solutions

The recent success in the US of methods advocated by physicians such as Dr Dean Ornish, which have received enormous publicity, shows that a combination of dietary change, the adoption of stress-coping strategies such as meditation and yoga, and the regular application of physical exercise within the tolerance of the individual can dramatically change cardio-vascular health, often restoring high blood pressure to normal while also reducing the chances of a heart attack enormously. *(See Chapter 3 for more on this.)*

Each of these approaches – dietary modification, stress-reduction and exercise – have long been known to influence hypertension. However it is only recently that evidence, proof positive, has been produced in long-term studies of the vast benefits of combining these approaches.

Each method helps, but together they help far more than the sum of their individual benefits – and this is to a large extent the message of this book.

Factors Negatively Associated with Hypertension

Having high blood pressure is a major danger to life itself under any circumstances. It carries the risk of wider ill-health affecting the heart, circulatory system, brain, etc. But having high blood pressure under specific circumstances, as listed below, increases these risks even more.

Some of these associated factors can be altered, others cannot, but they should at least be understood and the knowledge used as a means of focusing more strongly on those elements which can be changed.

Amongst the most important factors associated with serious ill-health being associated with high blood pressure are the following, most of which can be modified by means of strategies discussed later in this book.

- High cholesterol levels – something which can be altered over time by changing the diet, stress-reduction, exercise and specific nutritional and herbal treatment (and medication)
- Being overweight – which can also be altered or modified by the same methods
- Having a tendency to diabetes – also easily influenced by diet, exercise, stress-reduction (and medication)
- Being male, being black and being young (with a combination of these being even more serious)
- Being a smoker, the treatment of which may be difficult but which is essential if hypertension is to be controlled
- Having diabetes – which can be helped by diet, stress-reduction, exercise, supplementation and medication
- Having other organs already diseased – such as the kidneys or heart – which may make the application of dietary or lifestyle changes more complicated, but does not rule them out
- Having a persistently high diastolic pressure (the lowest of the two figures, taken which represents

the pressure achieved by the pumping heart) – which is far more serious than a persistently high systolic pressure. A high diastolic pressure can also be changed by means of diet, exercise and relaxation methods – as Dr Ornish's studies have proved within the last few years.

Hypertension is a disease of civilization and it is in the habits of a 'civilized' life that causes are to be found, and therefore answers as well.

Drugs and Hypertension

Usually a doctor will check blood pressure on a number of different occasions, and will satisfy him- or herself that the pressure is regularly high, before prescribing medication. An increasing number of doctors are suggesting methods which mirror some of those advocated in this book (and by Dr Ornish) before deciding (if results are not seen) to prescribe a combination of anti-hypertensive drugs. Many prescribe both dietary, lifestyle and stress-reduction approaches as well as drugs. However too many still prescribe medication without diet and lifestyle advice being offered, and many over-prescribe medication, despite evidence that, over time, this is a harmful approach.

There are a number of different ways in which drugs can modify pressure. Should drugs be employed in the treatment of high blood pressure they may fall into one of the following categories (a combination is usual):

- Centrally acting drugs – these act on the brain's mechanism for controlling the diameter of the blood vessels (obviously it is easier for the heart to pump blood through an open tube rather than one which is narrow).
- Beta-blockers – these reduce the force with which the heart pumps.
- Diuretics – increase elimination of urine through the kidneys, lowering the level of fluid in the body and therefore the amount of blood that needs pumping.
- ACE inhibitors – also assist in widening the diameter of the blood vessels, making it easier for the heart to pump blood, by acting on enzymes which influence this.
- Calcium channel blockers – ease the pressure on the blood vessels from the smooth muscles which surround them, so reducing the narrowing influence this can have on the vessels.
- Sympatholytic drugs – act to stop 'stress' messages from reaching the blood vessels by interfering with the sympathetic nervous system's transmission of information to the tissues which can constrict in response to stress.

ACE (angiotensin-converting enzymes) inhibitors/ Calcium channel blockers/Sympatholytics

These different classes of drug all act, in different ways, to produce vasodilitation, an 'opening' of the blood vessels, by lowering the pressure from the muscles which surround them. This effect therefore also reduces the pressure required to pump blood through the blood vessels and usually leads to an improved oxygen supply, something helpful in conditions such as angina where the heart muscles themselves become oxygen-depleted because of poor blood supply.

The ways in which these drugs work differ: the calcium channel blockers act directly on the muscles; the ACE inhibitors interfere with the enzyme activity in the blood which 'tenses' muscles; and the sympatholytics block nerve messages which would tense the muscles.

Side-effects

Quite obviously these drugs will also produce influences on areas and tissues which are not directly connected with the circulation and heart, and so side-effects are to be expected. These side-effects include flushing, headaches, dizziness, fainting and a build-up of fluid which could produce swollen ankles, for example.

A major danger exists of producing too low a blood pressure, and so the introduction and monitoring of the use of such drugs (there are many different forms of each class of these medications) is important.

Diuretics

These speed the elimination of fluid from the body. As excessive fluid in the body is turned into urine and eliminated, so does the work rate of the heart diminish, with less fluid to pump and with lower pressure in the blood vessels.

There are several parts and functions of the highly complex activity of the kidneys which are acted on by different diuretics – although the end result is much the same:

* osmotics prevent reabsorption in the kidneys of sodium and water
* potassium-sparing diuretics do much the same but prevent loss of potassium salts
* thiazides – the most widely used diuretics in treating hypertension – prevent reabsorption of water, sodium and potassium, and so are often prescribed along with a potassium supplement
* Loop diuretics also prevent reabsorption of water, sodium and potassium but in different ways from any of the other drugs, acting very rapidly and strongly and so used very selectively in special circumstances.

As fluid elimination is increased in these ways, tissues which were previously swollen should normalize.

Side-effects

In many cases these drugs cause raised cholesterol and
uric acid levels – which can trigger gout; glucose intol-
erance (causing problems for diabetics); sexual dysfunction and imbalance in the potassium levels in the
body, leading to weakness and confusion and, at times,
heart irregularities. The potassium loss caused by
these drugs is usually balanced by taking extra supplements of this vital substance. General chemical imbalances may occur.

Beta Blockers – Adrenergic Antagonists

These are a range of drugs which act in a variety of
ways to influence the function of adrenaline, thus
influencing circulation and blood pressure. They
interrupt the reception of noradrenaline, which com-
mences in the adrenal glands and which has many
powerful influences around the body. For example, the
influence on blood pressure is due to a reduction in the
rate and the force with which the heart pumps blood.
It is because so many parts of the body are influenced
that the variety of potential side-effects is so large.

Side-effects

These include major breathing difficulties, poor circulation to the hands and feet, headaches, palpitations,
weakness, dry mouth, asthma, bizarre dreams, fatigue,
insomnia, sexual dysfunction, raised cholesterol levels,

or lower levels of the beneficial parts of cholesterol (high-density lipoprotein).

Low blood pressure can result from some forms of adrenergic antagonists; great care has to be taken by monitoring the use of these drugs.

Altogether the field of drug therapy for high blood pressure is littered with the names of once-popular drugs which have been withdrawn as a result of unacceptable side-effects.

This is not really surprising, since the aim of each of these drugs, in its own way, is to alter one or other aspect of the complicated circulatory system with a view to lowering the blood pressure. Whilst frequently achieving that goal, there is in each and every case a degree of side-effect apparent as the system tries to cope with the alterations forced upon it by the drug. The very nature of high blood pressure makes it likely that anything forcefully altering aspects of the body's physiology is bound to have repercussions throughout the body.

Blood pressure is a function. High blood pressure is a function which is exaggerated as the system attempts to cope with unusual or undesirable factors. To alter, using drugs, the blood pressure, without in some way attempting to deal with the causes of its elevation, is to court disaster.

This is not to say that, in extreme cases, there is not a good case for the employment of one or other of these drugs, at least in the short term. This does not in any way excuse the avoidance of dealing with causes, which must precede any real control or return to normality of a blood pressure which is high.

There is a growing awareness amongst medical researchers and practitioners of the need for greater attention to causative factors, as well as to non-pharmacological methods such as those outlined in this book. These include weight reduction, salt limitation, stress-reduction methods, moderation of alcohol and tobacco usage, appropriate levels of cardio-vascular exercise, behaviour modification (quitting smoking, for example) and dietary changes.

The medical attitude to these methods seems to be that whilst they hold great promise and should be used whenever appropriate, they do not take the place of drug control. This may be a fair comment where pressure is so high that it endangers life. Combining drug treatment alongside non-drug self-help approaches would then seem to be the best choice. In the field of prevention and dealing with mild hypertension, the non-drug methods have been shown to be superior, since they deal with causes and not symptoms, and they are, without exception, safe.

No advice contained in this book should be taken as advice to avoid medical care. Awareness of alternatives and of the inherent dangers in drug methods should lead to an intelligent and co-operative involvement in the programme to recover and to maintain health at its optimum level, as well as preventing ill-health, including high blood pressure.

We will now examine more closely some of the major causes of hypertension.

3
The Causes of High Blood Pressure

Stress

Stress is probably the most easily demonstrated cause of increasing blood pressure. Whenever we are under stress, upset, angry, anxious or called upon to adapt to unusual conditions or situations, the body responds by preparing for activity by co-ordinating a variety of rapid internal changes. Among the most important of the changes which take place almost instantaneously after any such challenge is the release of the hormone adrenaline by glands which lie above the kidneys. This, and other secretions, cause the blood vessels to narrow, aiding in the rapid transmission of oxygenated blood to the muscles and brain. This is also achieved by increasing the heart rate and, naturally enough, by a rise in blood pressure. Arousal of this sort is a normal physiological response to the demands of life. Unfortunately though, in modern life such demands can become repetitive or even constant. In such a situation the rise in blood pressure and the narrowing in diameter of the blood vessels can also be an almost constant factor. If blood pressure is already higher than normal, then such additional increases can be severely compromising for the body and can result in a cerebral accident (stroke) due to a failure of one of the blood vessels to cope with the increased strain of high pressure. In any case, the rise in blood pressure via stress factors can be seen to be a major cause of chronic hypertension.

Learning to avoid arousal, anger, anxiety and other forms of obvious emotional stress is therefore of some importance to anyone repetitively affected in this way. The application of de-stressing methods, including relaxation and meditation techniques, or of biofeedback methods is often helpful, and this will be discussed in later chapters. It should be clear, though, that each individual cause of high blood pressure is seldom found to be acting alone; more commonly there will be a number of interacting elements making up the complex picture.

Salt

Salt may be one such additional factor. This has been shown in many individuals to have the ability to upset the delicate biochemical balance that exists in the body between sodium (a constituent of salt) and potassium. It is known that in areas of the world where salt intake is high there is also a tendency for high blood pressure to be prevalent. Among many population groups where the salt intake is below 500 mg a day, there is often a tendency for blood pressure to fall rather than rise with advancing age. The converse has also been noted. Indeed, in one group of South Sea Islanders who cook their vegetables in sea water and ingest as much as 15,000 mg of salt daily, the blood pressure of all people, including children, was elevated.

There is, however, known to be a degree of individual susceptibility. This susceptibility is also known to be greater in young people, so that a high salt habit started in infancy may be seen to be laying the foundations for high blood pressure in later life. Although subsequent restriction of salt is seldom enough to return blood pressure to normal, it does improve the picture to some extent. It seems that high intakes of sodium, in salt, have a depressing effect upon potassium levels. These two minerals interact in a close manner in the transport of nutrients to the cells, and the discharge of wastes from the cells. Anything which dramatically alters the relationship between them also alters the dynamics of cellular physiology with grave repercussions. A tendency can develop for extra-cellular fluid to build up, and this manifests itself in the body generally as swollen areas. This creates an extra degree of pressure on the tiny blood vessels and thus influences blood pressure as a whole. The usual medical treatment of such a situation is to use diuretics, which will 'flush' extra fluid from the body via the kidneys. This is at best a short-term measure since it does nothing to alter the reasons for the imbalance (although some diuretics include additional potassium to prevent further imbalance).

The prevention of high blood pressure would therefore seem to call for the avoidance of a high salt intake in infancy, and the moderation of its use generally. This is the safest advice, since although some people can obviously eat salt with impunity, there is no way of knowing to whom this applies until evidence of its harmlessness in the body is deduced by the maintenance of normal blood pressure into old age. Cutting down salt in existing cases of hypertension can certainly help to mitigate against the condition getting worse, and can help in the reduction of excessive levels. However, on its own, salt reduction will seldom allow a return to normal pressure. It should be seen as just one of a number of interconnecting factors in a programme to restore normality.

Associate Professor Melvyn Werbach, MD, of the University of California at Los Angeles, has researched nutritional influences on ill-health for many years. He reports that the balance of the diet, as far as four key minerals are concerned, has a major influence on blood pressure. These four minerals are: calcium, magnesium, potassium and sodium (found mainly in salt). He quotes many research studies which show that restricting salt (ideally to less than 1 gram daily) in people already affected by high blood pressure causes a reduction in approximately 60 per cent of cases. However, if no reduction has been noticed after two months of salt (sodium) restriction, this is probably not a factor in the condition.

He also shows clearly that supplementation of the diet with the other three nutrients mentioned (calcium, magnesium and potassium) – or altering eating habits to include food which provides these – as well as reducing sodium is a far more reliable approach. This highlights the need for a comprehensive approach to hypertension, rather than odd changes being made in the hope that this will correct what is a chronic problem with many factors interacting in its cause, progress and, therefore, in its resolution.

Smoking

Smoking is another common habit which has a direct and often dramatic effect upon blood pressure. The systolic pressure can rise by as much as 25 mm/Hg within seconds of the first puff of a cigarette (or pipe, or cigar). Once again this is because of the production by the body of adrenaline and, as in the stress example discussed above, the repetitive nature of the insult is what causes progressive damage.

Any smoker will notice that, in time, the circulation to the extremities will become impaired, and cold hands and feet will be common. This is evidence of the restricting effect upon the blood vessels, and the obvious result of this is to send blood pressure upwards as the body fights to get blood through narrower channels. Often such narrowing can lead to complete obliteration of the circulation to a limb, and the result of this may be gangrene, requiring amputation.

In less dramatic ways the average smoker can destroy normal function and increase blood pressure steadily over a long period of time. The combination of a highly stressed individual who also smokes can be seen to be a prototype for the hypertensive individual who is a candidate for an early coronary or stroke. Both factors, stress and smoking, are capable of being altered and the condition normalized, thus avoiding the ultimate disaster.

Eating Meat

Eating meat has been shown to increase blood pressure.

Many studies have been made of different groups of people with various dietary habits, and their health conditions, in relation to high blood pressure. Three examples are given below:

1 When two sets of around 100 people from two religious groups, one meat-eating (Mormons) and the other vegetarian (Seventh Day Adventists) were compared in 1984, it was found (after taking into account such factors as age, gender, height and weight, and alcohol and stimulant consumption) that on average both the systolic and diastolic pressures of the vegetarians were approximately 5 mm/Hg lower than those of the meat-eaters.

   Analysis of the diets showed that the vegetarians were eating significantly more unsaturated fat, fibre, vitamin C, vitamin E, magnesium, calcium and potassium, as well as far less cholesterol-inducing foods than the meat-eating group.

2 In another research project, 60 healthy meat-eating individuals were divided into two groups. One followed a vegetarian diet for two weeks and then reverted to their usual pattern, while the other group ate their normal diet for the first two weeks and then switched to a vegetarian diet (which included eggs and dairy foods) for another six weeks. The results showed that when switched to a vegetarian diet all participants showed a drop in blood pressure (approximately 5 mm/Hg systolic and 3 mm/Hg diastolic). These benefits were lost

when the subjects returned to their normal meat-eating diet. The amount of fat consumed was thought to be the key difference between the two diets.

3   In a different research study, approximately 100 confirmed adult vegetarians were compared with a matched group of non-vegetarians, living in the same urban environment. The average blood pressure of the vegetarians was 126/77 mm/Hg; that of the meat-eaters, 147/88. There was a significantly lower blood pressure in all age groups in the vegetarian group, and only 2 per cent of the vegetarians had high blood pressure (over 160/95) as compared with 26 per cent of the meat-eating group. The family history of high blood pressure was similar in both groups, and weight similarity was taken into account in all comparisons. The main difference between the groups, as far as individual nutrients were concerned, was found to be the much higher intake of potassium amongst the vegetarians which, as discussed in the review of the influence of salt on hypertension, is thought to be the significant factor in maintaining a lower blood pressure.

The vegetarians' diet was free of all meat and fish, and there were no more than three eggs eaten weekly, and hardly any dairy produce. The average pattern of eating was as follows:

Breakfast: Bread, fresh vegetables, yogurt or rice porridge

Lunch: Vegetable salad, boiled vegetables including potatoes or rice, pastries and fruits

Supper: Fresh vegetable salad with almonds, peanuts or nuts and fruit.

The fact that a sodium/potassium imbalance resulting from a high salt intake can result in high blood pressure, and that a diet rich in potassium (such as a vegetarian pattern as described) apparently has the opposite effect, gives us a clue as to the type of dietary pattern that would be helpful in both preventing and correcting high blood pressure. The recommended menus in this book (*see pages 110 and 112*) will not be entirely vegetarian, but will mirror the needs highlighted by this research.

Hardening of the Arteries

Also known as arteriosclerosis, this is the condition which many see as the main cause of chronic hypertension.

When the arteries become narrowed by the deposition on their walls of substances such as calcium, cholesterol, fibrin, etc. (known collectively as atheroma), the passage for blood becomes gradually reduced and the consequences are grave. Among the early symptoms is a rise in blood pressure to overcome the narrowed diameter of the arteries. This condition, which can itself be the major cause of further problems, is not able simply to arise in the body without predisposing causes. So although arteriosclerosis is a cause of high blood pressure, it is itself the result of biochemical alterations which may be the result of nutritional imbalances and deficiencies. It is obviously justifiable, and often essential, to tackle the existing concretions in the arteries by using a variety of means, some of which we will discuss; however the prevention of the condition is infinitely preferable.

One of the major causes of arterial damage of this kind is the activity in the body of a minute structure called a 'free radical'.

Free Radicals Explained

These are fragments of atoms or molecules which are created in the body in a cellular situation in which there is inadequate oxygen. The fragment is possessed of an unpaired free electron which allows the free radical to attach itself to an electron from any passing cell. This can start a chain reaction, because the particle which has lost its electron to the free radical automatically attempts to balance the situation by capturing the first available electron it comes across in turn. Thus the free radical can be seen to be a highly reactive and disruptive factor.

Its life may pass in a matter of a few thousandths of a second, yet the chain reaction it initiates may have vast repercussions involving many thousands of cells and molecules.

An example of 'oxidation' can be seen when an apple or potato is sliced in half and left in the open air: it will turn brown fairly rapidly. This is the oxidation process which we all take for granted. If the juice of a lemon is squeezed onto the exposed apple or potato surface, the browning is slowed or stopped. This is because lemon juice contains vitamin C – a powerful *antioxidant* which 'quenches' the free radical activity.

A similar process occurs when metal rusts (oxidation) or rubber perishes, or tissues in the body age and become wrinkled. It is also what happens when fats become rancid – which is almost exactly what happens in a small degree inside our bodies when there are too many fats and oils and not enough antioxidants.

Our own bodily defence systems (immune system) also produce free radicals as a means of killing invading bacteria and viruses, but in minute quantities which are prevented from doing any damage by the controls within the body. However, because the nutrients needed for this control are deficient (vitamin C, for example) or because there is just too much free radical activity (because of a high-fat diet, for example), control beaks down and damage occurs.

Should such a reaction take place in an artery, the resulting damage would affect the cells lining the walls of that artery. Cells in the artery wall can be induced, in this manner, to mutate, and this in turn results in the deposition in the damaged area of plaque, which is made of fibrin (blood protein laid down as a protective blanket) and also undesirable superfluous fats which may be present in the bloodstream such as cholesterol and triglycerides, and also calcium. Thus one cause of the formation of atheroma, and consequent narrowing and hardening of the arteries, is the free radical.

Predisposing Factors

Predisposition towards free radical damage may include the higher presence in the bloodstream of substances which can easily 'oxidize' or be affected by free radicals (*see below*).

Another key predisposing factor is the relative lack of antioxidant substances which mop up and destroy free radicals before they can do any damage. These include vitamins C and E (which research has shown – *see above* – to be far higher in the diet of vegetarians), as well as minerals such as zinc and selenium. There are also a number of amino acids which have this function, including methionine, cysteine and glutathione peroxidase. Vitamins B_1, B_5 and B_6 are also of assistance in controlling free radical activity.

When a relative lack of antioxidant nutrients is associated with exposure to pollution (cigarette smoke, alcohol, environmental pollution, etc.) or a diet high in factors which can degrade and form free radicals, such as fats and oils, then the likelihood of damage resulting from free radical behaviour becomes far greater.

High-fibre foods are one way of ensuring that free radical production is reduced, since such foods remove superfluous fats from the system. Much free radical activity begins with the breakdown products of foods in the bowel. The amount of time food residues spend in the bowel is important in this regard, since in the average Western bowel the transit time for food is between 75 and 100 hours, whereas the more 'primitive', high-fibre diet of other cultures produces a transit time of about 35 hours, with less, if any, free radical activity, and no atherosclerosis. This is also a key factor in the prevention of some major forms of cancer.

If we consider that the major demonstrable alteration leading to high blood pressure and heart disease is a degeneration of the arteries which carry fresh blood to the body as a whole and to the heart muscle itself, then the importance of free radical activity becomes clearer, as do the aspects of life which are conducive to free radical activity. These include a diet inadequate in essential antioxidant substances such as vitamins C, E, A, B_1, B_5, B_6 and zinc, selenium, etc., as well as a diet rich in fats, and an environment which contains pollutants and irritants such as smoke and alcohol (in excess).

Other Factors Contributing to Arteriosclerosis

There are a number of other identifiable factors which can be major contributors to the development of art-erial plaque deposits. One of these is chromium defi-ciency. Chromium is an important part of what is known as the Glucose Tolerance Factor (GTF). This is necessary for the production, and use by the body, of insulin, which controls the levels of sugar in the blood (*see 'The Sugar-Cholesterol Connection Explained', page 58*). If dietary chromium is low, and it usually is on a Western diet rich in refined carbohydrate products, then arteriosclerosis appears to develop more rapidly.

The precise relationship is not yet clear, but the fact is that there is a demonstrable lack of chromium in individuals who die of coronary disease. The best sources of chromium are yeast and black pepper.

Dietary Fats, Cholesterol and High Blood Pressure

Cholesterol is a vital part of the body economy, and 80 to 90 per cent of it is manufactured by the body itself. It is made in the liver and digestive tract from such food elements as sugars, proteins and fats. The 10 to 20 per cent of cholesterol in the body that is derived from the diet is therefore not the most important ele-ment in the situation. However, it is now known that how much cholesterol the body makes itself is also influenced by the eating pattern – notably by a high-sugar diet as well as other factors. This means that if there is a high cholesterol level (and this is of course highly undesirable because of the increased risks to the heart), then as well as finding ways of reducing the levels in the body and the amount being made by the body, there should also be some control over the intake of cholesterol-rich foods. The dietary pattern suggested later in the book (*see page 107*) will take care of all aspects of this requirement.

It is worth noting that cholesterol comprises a number of constituents, one of which, high-density lipoprotein (HDL), is in fact extremely beneficial. It acts as a scavenger of unwanted substances in the arteries and helps to protect against heart disease. Not everyone has high levels of HDL in their cholesterol; indeed some have an excess of low-density lipoprotein (LDL) – the harmful sort – instead.

Interestingly, one research finding has been that a moderate amount of alcohol intake (1½ glasses of wine daily) increases a certain form of HDL and this may act to protect against heart disease. Higher intakes of alcohol, however, are known to be harmful, leading to liver damage as well as to an increased risk of other degenerative diseases.

The aim of a diet which wishes to reduce the dangers of arterial damage, and so reduce the risk of heart disease and high blood pressure, must be to lower overall cholesterol levels to safe limits at the same time as increasing the proportion of HDL in that which remains.

It is worth noting that in young men between the ages of 16 and 27, the severe cystic form of acne which sometimes manifests itself is associated with a low level of HDL ('good' cholesterol), and that this can be seen as an early warning of cardiac problems which might emerge in years to come.

The process of damage to the arteries passes from the original free radical lesion, through the laying down of fibrin and the collection in the area of excess cholesterol and other blood fats, to a final stage in which calcification of the lesion begins. This involves the linking of the cholesterol deposits with calcium in an electrically charged attraction, which bonds like concrete. More fatty materials and calcium continue to build on to this structure, making the artery more rigid and narrower and consequently limiting the passage of blood and raising the blood pressure as a consequence.

The Sugar-Cholesterol Connection Explained

When you eat a carbohydrate – a starchy food – which is not used by your body as a source of energy (your body turns carbohydrate into glycogen – the fuel it burns to produce energy), the unused glycogen is stored. Storage capacity is limited, with some going to your muscles and a small amount – enough to meet the body's energy needs for a half a day or so – held in the liver.

What happens to the rest – to excessive amounts of consumed carbohydrate – bread, pasta, buns, sweets, juices?

Any carbohydrate eaten or drunk, over and above what can be stored as glycogen, is turned by the body into fat and deposited in the layers of the body where this is stored. This tendency to store carbohydrate as fat is even greater when the diet contains an abundance of simple sugars, because this triggers the pancreas to produce more of the main controlling substance which the body uses to deal with high sugar intake: insulin. Insulin removes excess sugar from the bloodstream and encourages its storage – as fat.

What Has This to Do with Cholesterol?

The liver is the main area of the body where cholesterol is manufactured. A particular enzyme (an enzyme is a minute but vital chemical substance used in body processes) called *HMG CoA reductase*, is what decides the rate at which cholesterol is manufactured in the body.

When excessive amounts of insulin are being produced by the pancreas in order to control excessive sugar levels in the blood, one of the by-products of this process is a stimulation of *HMG CoA reductase* – which means that more cholesterol will be produced – more than is actually needed.

High Sugar Levels – What Causes Them?

A high carbohydrate diet, especially one which includes simple sugars, will boost the levels of your blood sugar.

But so will anything which causes the adrenal glands to pump out adrenalin – which is the way the body prepares for action when stressed, and is another reason for keeping stress levels under review and using methods to help cope with these.

Adrenaline production – in response to stress – leads to sugar being released from the storage depots in the liver and muscles, so preparing the body to defend itself against danger.

When the adrenal glands are constantly or repetitively stimulated by stress to produce adrenaline – and therefore sugar – and if as a result blood sugar levels are repeatedly being made to increase, so causing the body to protect itself repeatedly from this by means of producing insulin, and if as a result even more *HMG CoA reductase* is produced – which stimulates cholesterol production – we can begin to see how stress can cause an aggravation of a high cholesterol condition.

If stimulants such as coffee and alcohol and cigarettes are regularly used – these also stimulate adrenaline and sugar production, and therefore *HMG CoA reductase*, and therefore cholesterol ... you can see the vicious cycle at work!

A low-sugar, low-stress, low-stimulant pattern can help all this. The dietary and other advice in this book aims to meet these needs.

The Fat-Cholesterol Connection

The fats in our diet – especially those derived from animal sources such as meat and dairy foods – are largely LDLs and undesirable.

The total amount of fat we consume adds to the cholesterol load in a direct way – the more fat you eat, the more LDLs there will be in the bloodstream.

A high-fat diet is linked in numerous research studies to atherosclerosis, venous thrombosis, strokes, heart attacks and, of course, high blood pressure – and as a result of these changes to a higher risk of death from these causes.

Saturated fats (solid at room temperature such as butter and margarine) are twice as powerful in raising serum cholesterol levels (and LDL levels) as are polyunsaturated fats (sunflower and safflower oils, for example), which should help in making choices as to how to cook and what to eat!

Dr Dean Ornish, Assistant Clinical Professor of Medicine at the University of California at San Francisco, has prescribed a combination of treatments –

mainly self-applied – to reverse atherosclerosis and hypertension.

This combination includes a vegetarian, low-fat and low-sugar diet, exercise, and stress-reduction methods including meditation and yoga – and his results are outstanding, far superior to any drug approach to these life-threatening conditions.

Some experts believe that the Ornish programme is successful for reasons other than those Dr Ornish himself believes. Lee Cowden, MD, an internationally renowned cardiologist from Dallas, Texas, believes that the key to the success of the Ornish programme is that the diet is low in specific protein fractions contained in meat, and high in vegetables and grains, which boosts vitamin and mineral levels (especially of the antioxidant nutrients) as well as containing fibre, which helps to eliminate excess cholesterol.

Bypass Surgery

When the blood vessels which carry freshly oxygenated blood from the lungs to the heart muscles become narrowed by the process of the build-up of calcium and cholesterol (atheroma), then the heart is in danger of oxygen starvation, and of a heart attack. This occurs when, through the narrowing process, the heart becomes starved of oxygen and some of it actually dies; or else a fragment of the atheromatous plaque breaks off and blocks the artery. By this time the individual will probably have had symptoms of angina (pain on exertion) for some time, as well as breathlessness. The current surgical procedure is to remove blood vessels from one of the limbs and graft these onto the heart so that they bypass the blocked arteries and carry fresh blood to the heart muscle.

Bypass surgery has become a major industry (an estimated $3 billion a year in the US). The results can be dramatic. However, in many cases the benefits are short-lived, and 50 per cent of these patients are dead within three years. The majority of the others are showing signs of silting up the new arteries by then, and the long-term prospects are not good. This is largely because of the failure of the individual to reform those aspects of his or her life which contributed to the problem in the first place.

An alternative method to surgery is being used by certain pioneering clinics in the US; this is called chelation therapy. This involves the use of a substance to remove from the arteries the calcified material which has obstructed them. It is accompanied by a programme of reformed nutrition to prevent recurrence. The decalcification of the arteries lowers blood pressure, as it removes one of the reasons for its increase. There are also a variety of natural methods of chelating calcium from the blood vessels; these will be outlined later (*see page 114*).

The dietary and exercise programme which will prevent and help to cope with high blood pressure will also be outlined later, but at this stage it is important to realize that most of the factors which lead to the degeneration of the cardio-vascular system, apart from inherited factors, lie firmly in the control of the individual. Some of the inherited factors can also be influenced, for example deficiency of vitamin B_6 in a pregnant mother can result in early changes to the blood vessels of her child, which can lead to athero-sclerosis later.

Among the chronic health problems which can, over a period of time, result in the development of high blood pressure, are conditions involving the kidneys and liver. As blood is obliged to pass through these organs on its circuit of the body, any of a wide range of ailments affecting them can influence blood pressure. It is not within the scope of this book to look compre-hensively at all these possible conditions, however it should be clear that if there is a major problem involv-ing the kidneys or liver then expert advice is required. If the general advice regarding nutrition, stress-reduc-tion and exercise is followed, then any tendency for minor dysfunction of the liver, in particular, should be eliminated. Kidney function will also be improved by following the same advice, but may require more specialized individual attention.

The liver is an organ which is easily affected by a less than adequate diet, especially one which includes exces-sive fats and refined foods, together with stimulants such as coffee, tea and alcohol. The reforms outlined in Chapter 5 together with periodic detoxification via fasting (*see Chapter 6*) will enable the liver to regenerate quite remarkably. There are also a number of specific aids that can be employed, such as amino acids, to speed detoxification of this most important organ. Some experts believe that general liver congestion resulting from nutritional imbalance and lack of exercise is one of the main reasons for high blood pressure.

The drinking of tap water, especially in cities and industrialized areas, is thought to produce additional strain on the kidneys due to the content of undesirable chemicals and contaminants. The use of a water filter on taps, or the substitution of spring or mineral water for tap water, are alternatives. Perhaps the best water of all is that derived from the cooking of vegetables. Once water has been boiled, chlorine, one of the harmful factors in tap water, will have been eliminated. The mineral content of water in which vegetables have been cooked is high. This has been called potassium broth, and it will be referred to in the chapter dealing with suggested foods. A fast on such a broth, or its use in regular eating patterns, is most valuable. It helps to balance the sodium-potassium ratio which, as we have seen, can be a cause of high blood pressure.

Some individuals also display calcium imbalance, which can be related to kidney problems. It is frequently found that an increased intake of calcium and vitamin C helps in the normalization of such problems. Such an imbalance may be accompanied by night-time cramps. Advice on quantities of supplements will be given later.

A connection has also been established between a dangerous form of hypertension which occurs in late pregnancy and calcium deficiency. The toxaemia of pregnancy includes high blood pressure as one of its symptoms. The addition of half a gram of calcium daily reduces the chances of this happening. Zinc is also deficient in such conditions, and experts believe that is linked to the calcium deficiency.

The interaction of many substances can be seen to be important, and this gives a clear indication that a balanced wholefood diet containing adequate quantities of all the vital nutrients is important, especially to the expectant mother. If these nutrients are unavailable through diet alone, then supplements can be used.

In general terms, high blood pressure usually results from a combination of stress factors, inadequate exercise and nutritional imbalance. The many ways in which different levels of these factors can manifest themselves in a variety of health problems, including high blood pressure, is evidence of the complexity of the human body.

Hypertension may result from different causes and so the approach to its normalization must vary. Similar causative factors in different people may result in different ailments. Generalization as to what will result from particular habits is unwise. A high-salt diet with a highly stressed lifestyle may produce quite different health problems in different individuals, whereas apparently identical symptom patterns may have quite different causes.

In order to correct the dietary pattern towards normal general trends requires analysis; similarly with stress patterns and lifestyle habits. The sets of questions in Chapter 4 will help you to do this.

You are unique, and the pattern you require to help you towards health is also personally unique to you. The broad pattern of our needs may be the same, but idiosyncratic requirements, which all of us possess, require attention if we are to achieve optimum health.

4
Assessing Your Dietary and Lifestyle Pattern

Nutritional Checklist

The aim of this series of questions is to assess your general awareness and implementation of the importance of correct nutritional practices.

The more 'Yes' answers in the first set of questions, the more need to reform your overall pattern of eating.

The ideal would be for all these answers to be 'No,' but this is unlikely.

Sometimes = not more than once a week
No = less than once a week
Yes = about four times weekly, or more

1 Do you eat refined (i.e. white) flour products?
2 Do you include sugar (any type) in your diet, or eat sweets?

3 Do you drink coffee, tea, chocolate or cola drinks?
4 Do you drink alcohol other than the equivalent of
   1½ glasses of wine or a pint of beer daily?
5 Do you eat foods containing any chemical
   additives (colouring, flavouring, etc.)?
6 Do you skip meals?
7 Do you pick at food between meals?
8 Do you eat more than 175 g (6 oz) of animal
   protein daily?
9 Do you eat convenience, ready-made foods such
   as instant mashed potatoes, TV dinners or tinned
   foods?
10 Do you add salt to your food?
11 Do you eat fried or highly seasoned and spiced
   foods?
12 Do you eat fatty meats, smoked or preserved foods?

The next series of questions should ideally all be
answered 'Yes'. Use the same method for classifying a
'Yes', 'No' or 'Sometimes' answer as described above
in answering these.

1 Do you eat fresh fruit?
2 Do you eat salad?
3 Do you insist on fresh vegetables (not frozen or
   canned) only?
4 Do you use herbs or garlic for flavouring food?
5 Do you ensure adequate fibre in your diet?

6 Do you eat whole cereal products (such as brown rice and wholemeal bread)?

7 Do you drink bottled rather than chlorinated tap waters?

8 Do you take a multivitamin or multimineral supplement or a vitamin C tablet?

9 Do you eat non-animal proteins such as seeds, nuts, pulses?

10 Do you eat breakfast?

11 Do you eat natural yogurt?

12 Do you believe that what you eat affects your health in a major way for good or ill?

Scoring

Score 2 points for each *Yes* answer

Score 1 point for each *Sometimes* answer

Score 0 for each *No* answer

Deduct the score of the second 12 questions from the score of the first.

An ideal total should be a minus number, or zero. Any score above zero indicates a need for reform; if the score is above 6 there is great need for attention to your diet.

The methods outlined in later chapters on dietary changes should be studied and followed, and the target should be to work towards 12 'No' answers in the first set of questions, and 12 'Yes' answers in the second set when you retest yourself in a few months' time.

Deficiencies

Deficiencies can be a major factor in allowing a decline in health which may accompany the onset of high blood pressure or cardio-vascular problems. All of the questions that follow concern the symptoms of possible vitamin, mineral, enzyme or amino acid deficiency. These symptoms can have other causes, but if there are a number of 'Yes' answers, then following the programme of dietary changes given in this book, as well as adjusting your dietary pattern to meet the requirements as outlined by the previous two series of questions, will result in a great improvement.

Are your nails ridged?

Do your nails break easily?

Do you have white flecks in your nails?

Do your gums bleed when you clean your teeth?

Do you get frequent mouth ulcers?

Do you have stretch marks in your skin?

Do you get cracks in the corner of your mouth?

Does strong light irritate you?

Are your eyes, mouth or nose dry?

Have you lost your sense of taste or smell?

Does your skin scale or flake?

Do you have a strong body odour?

Do your feet smell strongly?

Do you bruise easily?

Do you have difficulty in recalling your dreams on waking?

Lifestyle

The pattern of life that we live is of major importance in normalizing tendencies towards hypertension caused by stress.

The following series of questions should help to identify areas of your life which can be easily modified.

The first six questions should yield a 'No' answer, and the second eight a 'Yes'. Modify your behaviour and lifestyle accordingly if you wish to achieve this goal.

Do you work more than 5½ days a week?

Do you work more than 10 hours on a work day?

Do you take less than half an hour for each main meal?

Do you eat quickly and not chew thoroughly?

Do you smoke?

Do you get less than seven hours sleep daily?

Do you regularly listen to relaxing music?

Do you practise daily relaxation or meditation?

Do you take 30 minutes' exercise at least three times weekly?

Do you have a creative hobby (gardening, painting, needlework, music, etc.)?

Do you play any non-competitive sport or activity such as walking, swimming or cycling or attend a yoga or exercise class?

Do you try to have a siesta or short rest period during the day?

Do you have a regular massage or osteopathic attention, or practise yoga or Tai Chi at home?

Do you spend at least half an hour outdoors in daylight each day?

Hypertension Tendency

A tendency to high blood pressure may exist as a result of any of the factors elicited by the following series of questions:

Were you raised or do you live in a city environment?

Were you not breastfed as a baby?

Are you showing any signs of premature ageing (early grey hair, early wrinkling, etc.)?

Have you been overweight, other than for brief periods (more than 15 per cent above ideal weight)?

Have you a history of following a strict low-calorie diet?

Is there a family history of blood pressure, heart disease or diabetes?

Have you been on the Pill for more than a two-year period?

Do you eat meat daily?

Do you add salt to your food at table, or like salty cooked food?

Are you competitive, work to deadlines, easily irritated and/or ambitious?

You have a moderate tendency towards high blood pressure if:

- you are under 50 and have answered 'Yes' to five of these questions

- you are 50–60 and have answered 'Yes' to four of these questions

- you are over 60 and have answered 'Yes' to three of these questions

Higher scores increase the likelihood, while lower ones decrease it. This is a rough guide only, but is surprisingly accurate for most people.

The insights that the series of questions in this chapter can give should help to focus your attention on those factors which are within your control. Some are not, of course, for they are a matter of what has already happened. Overall, though, the majority of harmful influences that can mitigate towards high blood pressure and cardiac problems lie well within your control. We will move on to self-help methods in the next chapter.

Personality Factors

There is a great deal of evidence that people who display particular characteristics – known as 'Type A' characteristics – are more prone to cardio-vascular disease in general and high blood pressure in particular.

These characteristics are often learned as habits of behaviour, and can be modified. Some of the techniques of relaxation which will be outlined later will assist in this.

Type A Questionnaire

Answer 'Yes' or 'No' to the following questions:

Are you impatient, handling delay badly?

Do you walk, move, eat, speak quickly?

Do you consider yourself restless?

Do you feel anxious when you are not occupied with work?

Are you easily angered by people or events?

Do you work quickly rather than methodically?

Do you often find yourself doing more than one thing at a time?

Do you consider yourself a forceful, dominant personality?

Are you competitive, wanting to win?

Do you seek promotion and advancement, either socially or at work?

Do you crave peer and/or public recognition?

Do you set yourself and/or work to deadlines?

Are you time-conscious, always punctual?

Do you have any nervous tics?

Do you commonly find that your fists are clenched or your hands are moving, perhaps touching your face or smoothing your hair?

If you answered 'Yes' to seven or more of these questions, you are undoubtedly a 'Type A' personality, and as such more prone to cardio-vascular illness and hypertension than a 'Type B' who is characterized by the following traits – which many Type A people learn to mimic and adopt, often after their first coronary!

Type B Traits

patient; no anxiety felt if delayed

walking, moving, eating and talking slowly, without rush

happy to be idle

slow to anger, difficult to arouse

doing one thing at a time

retiring, easy-going, not pushy

not competitive at work or play

content with things as they are

not concerned with the opinion of others

happy to ignore deadlines

not time-conscious

relaxed (face and hands), composed

5
Self-help for High Blood Pressure

n this section we are going to examine a variety of self-help methods which can be employed safely at home by anyone. It must be re-emphasized, though, that these recommendations are not meant to take the place of expert professional advice, which should be sought if blood pressure or health problems are anything other than mild.

The methods presented all offer potential for general health improvement, and this is as it should be, since in the main the advice is aimed at improving the total body-mind complex which makes up each of us, with reduced blood pressure a by-product of such endeavours.

By improving our general function and by avoiding those factors which specifically, or generally, create the situation in which high blood pressure can manifest itself, the self-healing aspects of the body can come into play. This is a process (or more accurately a series of processes) which is known as homoeostasis.

Homoeostasis is something we take for granted – the mending of a broken bone, recovery from an infection and also the constant balancing of systems such as circulation and hormone secretion to meet the constant changes and needs of the body as a whole. Homoeostasis represents the body's constant striving for balance, normality and health, which is continuous throughout life. A stable blood pressure which varies with demands is one aspect of homoeostasis in action – standing up after lying down, for example, demands a change in blood pressure, as do all activities which exert us, and so a high blood pressure is evidence of homoeostasis in crisis, an attempt to maintain normality in unusual circumstances (narrowed arteries, for example).

In order to encourage a 'normal' homoeostatic response we need to replace bad habits with good ones, remove those obstacles to health which we can alter, and encourage the return to normality which will follow. Our attention in this objective will range through lifestyle and behaviour factors to exercise, breathing and relaxation methods, the use of nutritional supplements and dietary measures, all of which can be modified to help in the quest for health. Finally, we will also examine the most ancient of therapeutic measures, fasting, as a means of self-help towards normal blood pressure.

As demonstrated by the pioneering work of researchers such as Dr Dean Ornish, this is not just a hopeful quest but something which 'works'. What is on offer to anyone who feels that they can undertake the self-discipline involved is a series of dietary and lifestyle changes which can make a major difference to hypertension and cardio-vascular disease, both in terms of prevention and recovery.

Lifestyle and Behaviour Factors

You will have answered the questions in the self-assessment in Chapter 4 and this will have given you a first indication of some aspects of your lifestyle which may need attention. Such simple measures as ensuring that you get adequate rest and sleep, and that you modify any obvious stressful traits in the way you carry out your everyday duties and activities, are important and worth consideration, and possibly action.

We need adequate rest and sleep. Depending upon your particular needs, this can mean anything from six to eight hours daily. If you have not been giving attention to this vital aspect of your life, begin now.

An afternoon nap or siesta can also be a valuable aid, and many people find that this can be incorporated into their lunch break if they are at work. By having 20 or 30 minutes of complete rest at this time of day, a good deal of stress can be eliminated, and the rest of the day can be faced with renewed energy. If more time is available, then an hour or so of actual sleep or just rest with the eyes closed is ideal. Contrary to popular opinion, this sort of rest does not subsequently interfere with the night's sleep, but has actually been shown to enhance it. It also helps considerably in the overall lowering of what has been called 'arousal', which simply means increased tension. If you can learn a simple relaxation method (*see page 93*) then this could beneficially be carried out at such a time, to good effect.

Personality Type

Attention to adequate sleep and rest should be accompanied by some thought as to more general behaviour. As was noted in the questionnaire on personality in Chapter 4, some people are habitually in a hurry, always trying to do too many things and often doing more than one thing at a time ('Type A' individuals). Such people are often ambitious, competitive, quick-moving, quick-eating and quick-talking. There is also probably a tendency to work to deadlines and to be punctilious about time-keeping. Did you recognize any of these characteristics in yourself when you completed the questionnaire?

The evidence is strong that this sort of personality is far more prone to high blood pressure and cardio-vascular disease than the more relaxed, slow-moving 'Type B' personality. Many people have learned how to alter their behaviour from 'A' to 'B' by the simple method of concentrating on one aspect of behaviour at a time, say eating slowly or being less anxious about time-keeping, with great success. By 'copying' the behaviour which Type B people display it is possible to alter from one type (A) to another and to acquire the protection from stress-induced disease that this offers.

Unfortunately the decision to attempt to alter behaviour is often not made until a serious scare, such as a coronary, has concentrated the minds of both the individual ('Type A' behaviour is usually a male characteristic, although increasingly it is seen in women as well) and his medical advisers. The preventative modification of such behaviour is obviously desirable, and this can have a marked effect upon hypertension and general health over time. The adoption of creative, non-competitive hobbies, and regular, non-stressful exercise habits, preferably in the fresh air during daylight hours, as well as improving the sleep and rest factors discussed previously, all combine to create an atmosphere in which stress can be reduced and health enhanced.

Exercise

This is of course a key factor in reducing blood pressure, as well as improving heart and circulatory health.

It is vital that no one undertake vigorous exercise of any sort without first having a thorough check-up, and ideally an exercise tolerance test to assess how the heart and blood pressure react to exercise.

There is, however, one entirely safe form of exercise: walking. Everyone who can walk should do so, and should do so regularly and methodically. Thus, it is safe to say that at least 30 minutes should be spent walking, at least every other day. The speed and distance involved should be dictated by the conditions, terrain, etc. available, and the person's present health status. Ideally, walking should be on level ground, and the speed should be such as not to produce any distress at all. It should, however, result in a mild degree of heavy breathing.

There should be no suggestion of any sensation of pain, constriction or discomfort, in the chest, arms, neck, jaw, etc. during such walking. If there is, then medical attention is essential, as this may indicate that the heart muscles are inadequately supplied with blood. If however there is no such reaction, then a moderately brisk walk (not a jog, unless this is first cleared with your medical adviser) at the intervals mentioned (more if possible) can only help.

The long-term blood pressure response to such increased activity is to reduce it, since the increased efficiency of the circulatory system, as a result of the muscular activity, reduces the load on the heart and helps the veins to reduce their back-pressure. If possible, part of the walking exercise should be accompanied by one or other of the breathing exercises outlined later in this chapter.

Apart from walking, the use of a static bicycle, or swimming (in suitably warm water) are reasonable alternatives. Neither of these has the benefits of walking, however, and they are only mentioned as safe, rather than as equally desirable.

Aerobic Exercise

Put at its simplest, regular exercise which 'trains' the cardio-vascular system leads to a decrease in blood pressure, a reduction in the incidence of coronary artery disease and a lowering of overall cholesterol levels while actually also increasing the beneficial HDL levels.

For best results, then, exercise should aim to have an 'aerobic' effect – a cardio-vascular training influence – and to do this certain basic rules need to be followed.

- Have a check-up and get the all-clear to undertake regular aerobic exercise (if this is not carried out at least three times weekly for no less than 20 minutes at a time, results are likely to be disappointing).
- Now you need to calculate two figures – one is a level of heart activity (measured by pulse rate),

above which you need to go to achieve the aerobic effect. The other figure is the upper, safe limit of pulse activity above which you must *not* go during the exercise sessions.

- Deduct your age from the number 220 (the highest rate a healthy heart can ever safely reach). Let's say you are 50 years old. 220 - 50 = 180. This is the highest level your pulse should be allowed to go during exercise.

- Now calculate three quarters of this figure: 180 ÷ 4 = 45; 45 × 3 = 135. This the lowest rate of pumping at which your heart will start to benefit from exercise in an aerobic manner.

- To achieve full benefit, this rate (between 135 and 180) needs to be achieved for 20 minutes, three times weekly (i.e every other day).

- During exercise – walking rapidly, light jogging, using a treadmill exerciser at a gym or in the home – the pulse should be checked at least every five minutes to assess that the upper limit is not being passed and that the lower limit has been achieved.

- Obviously someone of a different age will have other target figures.

- As fitness increases, so the amount of effort needed to reach and sustain the training pulse rate will increase.

- Above all, check first that aerobic exercises are safe for you before commencing, and then try to maintain your commitment to performing them regularly. The benefits are proven.

- The method whereby the aerobic effect is achieved is of course optional, with jogging or treadmill walking the most popular and obvious. Many other choices exist, ranging from step exercises (under supervision ideally) to skipping with a rope, dancing or joining an exercise class.

Because of the likelihood of inducing a 'stress response', all competitive sport should be avoided for the duration of any anti-high blood pressure campaign.

Golf is sometimes suggested as a good way of getting some walking done. Its disadvantages include the tendency for a competitive edge to creep into it, as well as the fact that the walking involved is not continuous but is broken up into segments, with pauses to find, address and hit the ball. It is also frequently the case that golf courses are undulating, and a good deal of uphill walking is therefore called for. This may be undesirable.

Walking is always safe and extremely valuable, and essential as part of any programme for lowering blood pressure when it is high, and keeping it normal. Aerobics, if safe for you, are even better.

Breathing Exercises

The use of controlled breathing is another vital element in the programme. As mentioned in earlier chapters, the circulation of blood round the body is assisted by the major pump mechanisms of the muscles of the body as well as the activity (rise and fall) of the diaphragm as it moves during the breathing cycle.

The need to improve the mechanism of breathing is twofold: to assist in this dual pumping mechanism and to increase the amount of oxygen available for the blood. This latter consideration is important inasmuch as the role played by the blood as an oxygen-carrier can vitally affect the blood pressure. If tissues are inadequately oxygenated they send messages of distress, demanding more oxygen to be supplied. This leads to increased blood being pumped to meet the need, with all the consequences of strain on the heart and increased pressure. If this is happening against a background of tension on, or partial blockage of, the vessels carrying the blood, the consequences can be even worse.

Another key reason for the regular use of breathing exercises is the effect they have on arousal, the increase in activity of the sympathetic nervous system which stress produces. In Chapter 2 we discussed some of the drugs now commonly used in treating high blood pressure. One class of medication is the sympatholytic drugs – which act to stop 'stress' messages from reaching the blood vessels by interfering with the sympathetic nervous system's response to stress, which is to constrict, putting direct pressure on blood vessels and so increasing the pressure needed to pump blood through them. Since it is possible to lower 'arousal' (which is another way of describing the sympathetic nervous system's response to stress) by means other than drugs, in fact by means of relaxation and breathing exercises, then it is important in any attempt to reduce blood pressure to adopt such exercises and to use them regularly.

Breathing exercises are therefore an important part of the self-help measures involved in lowering the blood pressure naturally and safely. The following exercises should be used so that not less than two of them are practised each day, as well as the one specifically designed to be used with walking.

Exercise One

There are many exercises to help improve breathing but there is just one which has been shown in medical studies to effectively reduce arousal and anxiety levels. This is an exercise based on traditional yogic breathing. The pattern is as follows:

1 Having placed yourself in a comfortable (ideally seated/reclining) position, exhale FULLY through your partially open mouth, lips just barely

separated. This outbreath should be performed slowly. Imagine if you will that a candle flame is just about 15 cm from your mouth, and exhale in such a way as to not blow this out. As you exhale, count silently to yourself to establish the length of the outbreath. An effective method for counting one second at a time is to say (silently) 'one hundred, two hundred, three hundred, etc'. Each count then lasts about one second.

2   When you have exhaled fully, without causing any sense of strain to yourself in any way, allow the inhalation which follows to be full, free and uncontrolled. The complete exhalation which preceded the inhalation will have created a 'coiled spring' which you do not have to control in order to inhale. Once again, count to yourself to establish how long your in-breath lasts. The counting is necessary because the timing of the inhalation and exhalation phase of breathing is a major feature of this exercise.

3   Without pausing to hold the breath, exhale FULLY, again as before through the mouth, blowing the air in a thin stream (again you should count to yourself at the same speed).

4   Continue to repeat the inhalations and exhalations for not less than 30 cycles of in and out.

5   The objective is that in time (some weeks of practising this daily) you should achieve an

inhalation phase which lasts for 2 to 3 seconds while the exhalation phase lasts from 6 to 7 seconds – without any strain at all.

6   Most importantly, the exhalation should be slow and continuous. It is no use breathing the air out in two seconds and then simply waiting until the count reaches 6, 7 or 8 before inhaling again.

7   By the time you have completed 15 or so cycles, any sense of anxiety which you previously felt should be much reduced. Also if pain is a problem this should have lessened.

8   Apart from ALWAYS practising this once or twice daily, it is useful to repeat the exercise for a few minutes (about 5 cycles of inhalation/exhalation takes 1 minute) every hour if you are anxious or whenever stress seem to be increasing. At the very least it should be practised on waking and before bedtime, and if at all possible before meals.

Exercise Two

1   Stand upright.

2   Take a deep breath through your nose and bend slowly to the right, running your right hand down the outside of your right leg and raising your left arm above your head, so that your body stretches to the right.

3   As the movement is continued, more breath should be slowly drawn in.

4 Now bend slowly to the left, and allow your left
   hand to go down your left leg, and your right arm
   to come over your head, to lever your body over to
   the left.

5 During this movement, breathe out slowly through
   your mouth.

6 Continue in this fashion, breathing in as you
   bend to the right and out as you bend to the left,
   10 times.

7 The sequence of breathing should then be
   changed: breathing in as you bend to the left, and
   out when bending to the right.

8 Do this 10 times as well.

This exercise is designed to bring about increased
expansion of the side of the chest. It is an excellent
exercise to increase the drainage of the lungs and to
stimulate their eliminative functions.

Exercise Three

1 Stand erect with your hands on your spine at
   the level of your waist; your fingers should point
   towards the front of your body.

2 Close your mouth and take in air, in small
   amounts, as if sniffing a flower.

3 Continue to fill your lungs until no more can be
   taken. As you breathe in, bend your body
   gradually backward.

4 When your chest is full, expel the air slowly through your mouth, while at the same time bringing your body to a forward-bending position.

5 This exercise requires practice. Do this 10 to 15 times at least once a day.

Walking and Breathing Exercise

As well as performing at least two of the exercises as described above each day (and preferably all three, and ideally morning and evening), the following pattern can be adopted whilst walking.

1 As you walk, breathe in through your nose to a count of three, four or five steps, to fill your lungs. The number of steps you take as you inhale will vary with your speed of walking and your general condition. Above all it must be a comfortable, unstrained pattern.

2 Hold the breath for one or two strides and then exhale, still through your nose, to a count of two or three steps.

3 *Note* that when doing breathing exercises in a static situation (sitting, lying down or standing) the breathing-out phase of the cycle should take slightly more time than breathing in, but when in an active phase (walking, swimming, etc.) the reverse is true: breathing in should take longer.

4 This pattern of counting and breathing as you

walk should only be carried out for a minute or two at a time during your walk (that is, around 10 cycles of inhalation/exhalation) or until you find it difficult to maintain the rhythm.

5 Repeat several times during a half-hour walk.
6 As your fitness increases and your lung capacity improves, so you will be able to do more and more of this type of controlled breathing during exercise.

There is strong evidence of the value of the breathing exercise patterns as described in reducing stress levels and in helping to lower blood pressure. The key to success lies in doing them as described and in doing them regularly.

Relaxation Exercises

Relaxation exercises are most important in helping to bring stress down to acceptable levels by lowering levels of sympathetic arousal. One, at least, of the following should be employed each day for not less than 10 minutes; if blood pressure problems are evident, then twice daily is suggested. These should be done at a different time from the breathing exercises, and at a time when there is no likelihood of being disturbed. It is often useful to have a relaxation exercise follow on directly from the yogic breathing exercise (Exercise One described above).

Breathing and Repeated Sound Meditation

- Sit or lie down in a comfortable position in a suitable room and encourage a sense of heaviness as you focus on your body, area by area, in order to assess each area for obvious tension.
- Start by focusing briefly on the feet and pass slowly on to the lower legs, thighs, hips, buttocks, abdomen, lower back, chest, shoulders, neck, face, arms and hands.
- Do not overlook the muscles of the eyes and jaw. Many people screw up the eye muscles or clench the jaw habitually. If this is one of your traits, then pay particular attention to releasing these areas prior to continuing with the exercise.
- This movement of your mind from area to area should be only a brief survey, not lasting for more than a few seconds in each region.
- As each area is visualized, any obvious tension should be released.
- If you are not sure whether a muscle or area is relaxed, tense it for a few seconds and then let it go.

This brief but effective progressive muscular relaxation, area by area, prepares you for the exercise proper.

It is worth emphasizing that relaxation is a passive act. You cannot 'try' to relax, for this is a contradiction in terms. Relaxation is a letting go, a switching off, which ideally involves no effort.

The suggestion that areas where you are not sure of the state of tension or relaxation should be tensed prior to 'letting go' is designed to help to imprint on the mind the contrast between the two states – tension and relaxation. In this way, a gradual awareness will develop enabling you to sense tension as it arises and, most importantly, to release it during everyday activities. This is the basis of progressive muscular relaxation methods – a further example of which is given later in this chapter.

For the purpose of this particular exercise, the method outlined above is all that is required as preparation for the following breathing method.

- Having spent a minute or, at most, two in scanning through and 'letting go' of the obvious areas of tension in the musculature of the body, begin to breathe in and out through the nose.
- Passively pay attention to your breathing and, as you breathe out, say silently and slowly to yourself any one-syllable word.
- Breathe in and out at any comfortable speed. There need be no rush, nor is there any need to make the breathing particularly slow. The rhythm should be as natural and unforced as possible, not particularly deep or unusually shallow.
- You may well find that the rhythm will alter from time to time, or that periodically you will let out a

very deep breath or sigh. Just let it happen and do not attempt to control the rhythm or depth of the respiration – simply use it to time the repetitive, slow enunciation of a word or sound in your mind.

- Many people use the word 'one' for this purpose, but any short word will do. Remember it should be said (silently in your mind) as you breathe out. This should continue for about 10 minutes.

- After about 10 minutes of this exercise, stop repeating the word and simply allow the mind the luxury of doing nothing. Allow it to linger in the still, peaceful state to which you have drifted.

- Initially with the eyes closed and later with them open, spend at least two minutes in this state of inactivity.

- Slowly get up and resume your normal activities. (It is unwise to get up too quickly, as over-oxygenation from the breathing may result in short-term giddiness.)

A feeling of stillness and calm should eventually be felt. In some cases a sense of happiness and deep relaxation is quickly achieved – while in others there is only a gradual sense of being less stressed. In all cases where this type of exercise is performed as described, positive physiological changes will take place, irrespective of subjective feelings. In other words, there is a degree of stress-reduction whether or not you sense it from the outset, and blood pressure will drop.

Many people expect immediate and obvious changes. If they become disappointed as to this expectation they may lose the discipline required for the regular performance of these exercises. This is regrettable, for it has been positively established that the benefits of the exercises often begin long before there is any actual conscious awareness of improvement. Each individual will reap the benefits of these exercises at his or her own pace.

The repetition of the word which has been chosen may well be interrupted periodically by intrusive thoughts. When this happens do not feel irritated, simply resume the use of the word to coincide with exhalation.

Progressive Muscular Relaxation

This method involves the systematic, conscious relaxation of all the body areas in sequence.

The position for this exercise should be reclining – either on the floor or on a recliner-type chair. Ideally there should be no distracting sounds and the clothing worn should not constrict in any way. (A few cycles of deep slow breathing should precede the exercise.)

- Starting with the feet, try to sense or feel that the muscles of the area are not actively tense. Then deliberately tighten them, curling the toes under and holding the tension for 5 to 10 seconds. Then tense the muscles even more strongly for a further few seconds before letting all the tension go and sensing the wonderful feeling of release. Try to register consciously what this feels like, especially in comparison with the tense state in which you were holding the muscles.

- Progress to the calf muscles and exercise them in the same way. First try to sense the state the muscles are in, then tense them, hold the position, then tense them even more before eventually letting go. Positively register the sense of release. (In doing this to the leg muscles there is a slight danger of inducing cramp. If this occurs, stop testing the area immediately and move on to the next.)

- After the calf muscles, go on to exercise the knees, then the upper leg, thigh muscles, the buttocks, the lower and upper back, the abdomen, the chest, the shoulders, the arms and hands, and then the neck, head and face. The precise sequence is irrelevant, as long as all these areas are 'treated' to the tensing, the extra tensing, and then the release.

Some areas need extra attention. The abdominal region is a good example. The tensing of these muscles can be achieved in either contraction (i.e. a pulling in of the muscles) or by stretching (i.e. a pushing outwards of the muscles). This variation in tensing method is applicable to many of the body's muscles.

Indeed, at different times it is a good idea to vary the pattern, and instead of, for example, contracting and tensing a muscle group, try to stretch and tense it to the limit. This is especially useful in the muscles of the face, particularly in the mouth and eye region. Individual attention to these is important. On one occasion it would be desirable, for example, for the 'tensing' of the mouth muscles to take the form of holding the mouth open as wide as possible, with the lips tense. On a subsequent occasion, the 'tensing' could be a tight-pursed pressing together of the lips. If there is time available, both methods of tensing can be employed during the same exercise, especially in the areas you know to be very tense. The muscles controlling the jaw, eyes, mouth, tongue and neck are particularly important, as are the abdominal muscles, since much emotional tension is reflected in these regions, and release and relaxation of them often has profound effects.

There are between 20 and 25 of these 'areas', depending upon how you go about interpreting the guidelines given above; each should involve at least 5 to 10 seconds of 'letting go' and of passively sensing that feeling.

Thus, 8 to 10 minutes should suffice for the successful completion of the whole technique. This should be followed by several minutes of an unhurried return to a feeling of warm, relaxed tranquillity. Focus the mind on the whole body – try to sense it as heavy and content, free of tension or effort. This might be enhanced by a few cycles of deep breathing. Stretch out like a cat and then resume your normal activities.

Autogenic Exercise

The distinction between a relaxation exercise and a meditation technique is blurred at all times, but never more so than in autogenic methods, which are a blend of the two.

True autogenic exercises need to be taught by a special teacher or practitioner well versed in this excellent system. The modified method outlined below is based on the work of the pioneer in this field, Dr H Schultz.

At least 15 and ideally 20 minutes a day should be given to the performance of this method. At another time of the day this, or another relaxation method, should also be performed again. This routine should become a welcome, eagerly anticipated oasis of calm and peace in your daily programme. Stress-proofing without such periods of 'switching off' is unlikely to be successful.

The exercises involve the use of specific, internally (i.e silent) verbalized messages to focus awareness on a particular area. No effort is involved, but simply a passive focus on and awareness of any sensations or emotions which may result from each message.

Imagination or auto-suggestion has been found to have definite physiological effects. By combining a sequence of autogenic (i.e. self-generated) instructions with the passive, focused aspect of meditation techniques, a powerful method of self-help has been created to reduce arousal and induce lowering of elevated blood pressure.

- A reclining position should be adopted, with the eyes closed. External, distracting sounds should be minimized.
- The exercise starts with a general thought, such as 'I am relaxed and at peace with myself.' Begin to breathe deeply in and out. Feel the light movement of the diaphragm and feel calm.
- *Stage 1* – The mind should focus on the area of the body to which the thought is directed. Start by silently verbalizing 'My right arm is heavy.'
- Think of the image of the right arm. Visualize it as being completely relaxed and resting on its support (the floor, arm of the chair, etc.). Dissociate it from the body and from will-power. See the limp, detached arm as being heavy, having weight. After a few seconds, repeat the phrase 'My right arm is heavy.'
- This should be done a number of times until what you imagine to be a minute has passed, before proceeding to the right leg (for a minute of the

same focus) and then the left leg and finally the left arm. At each area, try to sense heaviness and maintain a passive feeling in the process.

- *Stage 2* – Again, begin with the right arm, focusing on it as you silently verbalize 'My right arm is warm.' Repeat this and pause to sense warmth in the arm or hand. Repeat this several times. The pause should be unhurried. To encourage this feeling of warmth it may be useful to imagine that the sun's rays are shining onto the back of the hand, warming it. The sensation of warmth spreads from there to the whole arm. Spend approximately one minute with this awareness and focus on warmth in the right hand (or arm).

- Proceed through all the same areas of the body as was suggested in Stage 1 (right foot/leg, left foot/leg and finally left hand/arm), pausing for some seconds at each to assess sensations which may become apparent. Such changes as occur cannot be controlled, but will happen when the mind is in a passive, receptive state. This exercise increases the peripheral flow of blood and relaxes the muscles controlling the blood vessels. It is possible to increase measurably the temperature of an area of the body using these simple methods.

- *Stage 3* – Focus attention on the forehead and sense a coolness, a calm relaxed feeling. Spend about a minute with the phrase 'My forehead is cool' and

then deliberately clench your fists, bend your arms and stretch them out and complete the exercise with the phrase 'I am alert and refreshed.'
• Breathe deeply, stretch and continue the day's activities.

During Stages 1 and 2, the time spent on each area should not be less than about half a minute: it is however quite permissible to spend two or three minutes focusing on any one part, especially if a desired sensation of heaviness or warmth is achieved. It will probably be found that the desired sensation is more easily sensed in one Stage than another, and that some areas seem more 'responsive' than others. This is normal. It is also quite normal for there to be no subjective appreciation of any of the verbalized sensations. Do not worry about this. Even if nothing at all is sensed for some considerable time, possibly months, there is a great deal actually taking place within the body as a result of the whole exercise. Persistence, patience and a total lack of urgency are all that is necessary for this method to lead to a decrease in muscular tension and a sense of calm and well-being.

A side-effect of this particular method is frequently experienced in terms of much-improved peripheral circulation – that is, an end to cold hands and feet, as well as lower blood pressure.

Biofeedback

Biofeedback is a system which utilizes the 'feedback' to the individual of biological information not usually available to him or her, thus enabling the person to learn to exercise control over organs and functions which are normally outside voluntary control. By means of these techniques, individuals have achieved control over circulatory functions – as evidenced by the ability to increase the temperature of a particular body area. Other examples include control of the heart rate, blood pressure, gastric secretions, brain wave patterns, skin resistance to electricity, relaxation of muscle groups and so on. The effects of this system are profound, since such control has previously only been achieved using drug therapy.

The simplest biofeedback equipment is that which measures the electrical skin resistance (ESR). Electrode pads are attached to the palm or fingers of either hand. The information derived via the electrodes is fed into a machine; this, in turn, produces a sound which is louder when the ESR is low (indicating anxiety or tension), and softer when it is high (indicating calm and relaxation). The objective is to use the mind to silence the machine. This is achieved by trial and error until the individual learns what to do to reduce the sound level completely. At this point a relative state of relaxation will have been achieved. The control of blood pressure and heart rate can be achieved in a similar way.

What is not certain is whether, in the long term, the individual, having 'learned' to achieve the desired result whilst attached to biofeedback equipment, can continue to do so in everyday life. Other systems, such as meditation and relaxation techniques, have the ability to influence everyday experience as well as allowing the possibility of increased 'awareness' and personal development. Biofeedback cannot, as yet, make similar claims. The best results with biofeedback have been achieved when such methods are combined with meditation and relaxation exercises such as autogenics, as described above.

Simple biofeedback equipment to monitor ESR or skin temperature can be purchased for very reasonable amounts. No explicit instructions as to what to do to achieve the desired result, whether it be raising or lowering the temperature, or raising the ESR, are provided. The essence of the technique is for the individual to learn by repetition what it is that has to be done, using the mind to alter the sound being given off by the machine or to switch off the light on the machine. It is a system which requires internal experimentation and, initially, the results might well be chaotic, as noises get louder in response to 'wrong' signals, for example.

Nutrition

Nutrition is the major key to reducing high blood pressure, and it is this area which calls for your most dedicated efforts. You will find set out the key factors in the diet which are undesirable as far as building up problems which can result in hypertension. These include refined products (white flour, sugar, etc.) and fats which contribute to free radical activity and consequent damage to blood vessel walls, as well as resulting (with refined foods) in overweight, a major factor in hypertension development.

Fats of course also add to the substances which become part of the clogging process in the arteries. Eating excessive quantities of meat has been shown to be a key factor, as has the use of sodium-rich foods, especially salt (in certain people). The consumption of alcohol should also be modified.

This leaves a diet in which the foods that need to be emphasized as being helpful include the low-fat proteins such as fish, poultry (not the skin, though) and low-fat cheese; all vegetables and fruits, and the whole range of grains, seeds, nuts (unsalted and not roasted) as well as all the pulse family (beans of all sorts), with all the wonderful flavours and textures that this offers.

The dietary pattern outlined below should be adopted over a period of several weeks, rather than overnight. The closer you can get to it, the better. Not all foods are suitable for all people, and tastes differ greatly. Within the general outline and choices described there is ample opportunity for finding an individual pattern. At the end of this section you will find notes on fasting. The use of simple short fasts (24 to 36 hours), as well as the occasional two- or three-day fast, helps enormously in preparing the body for the detoxification and regeneration which is so vital to renewed health and vigour and recovery of cardiovascular efficiency.

The following are general dietary guidelines followed by a list of foods to avoid (with suggested alternatives), and then an outline of a menu which can be adapted to your own needs and tastes.

General Rules of Eating and Diet

1   Digestion begins in the mouth. Food should be eaten slowly and chewed thoroughly.
2   Avoiding foods that are very hot or very cold will improve digestive functions.
3   Drinking any liquid with meals interferes with digestion, as does any liquid taken up to an hour after a main meal.
4   Simple meals without sauces are easier to digest. Combinations of certain foods can produce indigestion – for example, protein and carbohydrate do not mix well (bread and cheese or fish and chips).

5   Fried and roasted foods are difficult to digest and
    should play little or no part in the diet.

6   *Foods to Avoid:*

    All white flour products, such as white bread,
    cakes, pasta, pastry, biscuits. Replace with
    wholemeal alternatives.

    All sugar of any kind and its products, such as
    sweets, jams, soft drinks, ices, etc. Replace with
    fruit, dried fruit, sugarless jam, fresh fruit juice,
    fruit-flavoured natural yogurt, etc.

    Polished (white) rice. Replace with unpolished
    (brown) rice.

    Any foods containing additives, preservatives,
    colouring, etc., such as most tinned and prepacked
    foods.

    Tea, coffee, chocolate. Replace with herb teas,
    dandelion or other coffee substitutes.

    Strong condiments (vinegar, pickles, pepper,
    curry, etc.). Replace with herbs.

    Milk, butter, cream and their derivatives. Use
    only low-fat cheese in moderation, natural yogurt
    or sour milk (*acidophilus* milk).

    Margarine.

    Salt and salted foods.

    Meat. If animal protein is to be eaten, then fish
    and chicken (no skin), etc. are more desirable than
    red meat. Eat no more than four eggs weekly.

7 *Foods to Include:*

Drinks: Herb teas (red clover, spring water, sage, camomile, etc.). Coffee substitute (Pioneer, carob, dandelion). Fresh unsweetened fruit juice and vegetable juices. Nut/soya milk.

Cereals: Millet, oatmeal, unpolished rice, buckwheat, barley, rye or wholemeal bread, sprouted grains (wheat).

Proteins: Fish, chicken, liver, occasional lean meat.

Beans: Chickpeas, lima, soya, lentils, etc.

Sweeteners: A little honey, date sugar or maple syrup.

Fruits: Apples, bananas, pears, avocados, cherries, apricots, peaches, nectarines, papaya – if possible organically grown and unsprayed. Dried fruit (if sun-dried).

Nuts: Walnuts, almonds, pecans, hazelnuts, unsalted peanuts.

Vegetables: All fresh or freshly frozen vegetables.

Seasoning: Parsley, chives, garlic, sage, mar-joram, thyme, oregano, powdered kelp, vegetable seasoning (without salt). Salt substitute such as potassium chloride.

Seeds: Sunflower, pumpkin, sesame, apple, nectarine, pear.

Sprouting seeds and beans: Mung beans, wheat sprouts, alfalfa, etc. Include these in salads or use as a sandwich filler.

Soups: Include any vegetables, plus beans, millet, cereals (no meat or fat stock).

8 *Undesirable Foods* (if cardio-vascular health is to be improved):

Tap water (high in heavy metals such as cadmium and lead, which provoke free radical activity).

Tea, coffee, alcohol, bottled soft drinks.

Processed cereals (i.e. flaked, puffed, etc.).
All white flour products.

Fat meat, bacon, pork, ham, tinned or smoked meat, salted meat.

Cane or beet sugar, artificial sweeteners.

Butter, full-fat milk, cream, full-fat cheese.

Tinned fruit, sulphur-dried fruit.

Roasted or salted nuts or peanuts.

Tinned vegetables.

Salt, pepper, curry, chilies, etc.

Salted or roasted seeds.

Tinned, packet or block soups.

General Menu Sheet

Breakfast
Choose from:

1 Oatmeal porridge (without salt or sugar) and honey if desired.

2 Muesli (oats, nuts and dried fruit mixture) moistened with fruit juice, soya milk or natural yogurt. Add a little honey if desired.
3 Wholemeal bread or toast. Yeast spread or sugarless jam.
4 Fresh fruit and/or soaked or lightly cooked dried fruit (no sugar). Drink herb tea or coffee substitute or fresh fruit juice.

Breakfast is a very important meal in balancing the body's metabolism and should not be skipped.

On three days a week have a boiled or poached egg for breakfast as well if you fancy this.

Midmorning
Fresh fruit or rice cakes or sunflower/pumpkin seeds or unsalted nuts and/or herb tea.

Lunch
Ideally this meal should be mainly a salad meal. If it is not, then the evening meal should contain a large mixed salad. Use as many ingredients as are in season. Dress with lemon juice and olive oil and a little cider vinegar (no other vinegar or salt).

Add wholemeal bread or a brown rice savoury, or a baked potato (in its skin). A small amount of low-fat cheese may be added, but it should be remembered that this meal is meant mainly to be a salad and carbo-hydrate meal.

Evening Meal

This meal should mainly be protein such as fish or chicken (not the skin) or liver or, no more than once a week, red meat (lean) or a vegetarian combination of pulses (beans) and cereals (such as brown rice). Add to this fresh vegetables or salad.

Dessert

Fresh fruit.

This pattern of eating should be followed for not less than six months in order to achieve a degree of control of blood pressure. Do not expect results inside the first two months. Results will come but the reversal of a major trend towards ill-health does take time, and you must give the body a chance. When a reasonable level of blood pressure is achieved, the knowledge gained by this whole exercise in self-help will enable you to maintain it, by adapting the diet and relaxing only slightly the dietary pattern described above.

Supplements

These are known to be helpful in reducing blood pressure and to assist cardio-vascular function. Include the following:

- Vitamin C with bioflavonoids – 1 g daily
- Vitamin E (d-alpha tocopherol) – 200 to 400 iu daily

- Vitamin B complex – a formula which contains at least 25 mg each of vitamins B_1, B_2, nicotinamide (B_3), calcium pantothenate (B_5) and pyridoxine (B_6) – 1 daily
- As an alternative to this, 8 brewer's yeast tablets can be taken daily.
- Magnesium orotate – 500 mg daily
- Potassium orotate – 150 mg daily
- Manganese orotate – 50 mg daily
- Selenium – 50 micrograms daily
- Garlic capsules – 2 daily (very helpful indeed in blood pressure treatment)
- Bromelaine enzymes (pineapple derivative) – 1 200-mg tablet twice daily before food
- Glutathione (amino acid compound) – 500 mg twice daily

Glutathione is an amino acid combination which assists in the removal of free radicals from the system. It, and the other supplements listed, are totally non-toxic at these dosages.

The B_{13} minerals (orotates of magnesium, potassium, etc.) as well as the bromelaine enzymes and glutathione can be obtained from most health food stores.

Chelation
Deposits of calcium in the arteries can be removed by the oral route as well as the more efficient, but more

difficult, intravenous method discussed in Chapter 3. The following is an outline of the pattern of supplementation recommended by Dr Morton Walker and Dr Garry Gordon in their book *The Chelation Answer* (Evans, 1982). They suggest a variety of nutrients which interact to chelate cholesterol and calcium deposits out of the arterial walls. Taking such high levels of supplements should be achieved over a period of several months, and should not be started immediately at full dosage. Begin with about a quarter of the dosages recommended, and slowly build up to the required level, maintaining this for six months or so.

The dietary pattern outlined previously should be maintained throughout this programme, together with exercise and other recommendations. **These supplements should replace those suggested above, not be in addition to them.**

Oral Chelation Programme (ultimate daily requirement):

- Lecithin – 4 g
- Wheatgerm (source of vitamin E) – 1 tablespoon
- Evening Primrose Oil – 500 mg (or 12 g sunflower seeds) as a source of linoleic acid
- Vitamin C – 4 g
- Niacin (vitamin B_3) – 50 mg, three times daily

- Vitamin B_{15} (also known as dimethylglycine, DMG) – 250 mg
- Vitamin B complex – 1 strong tablet
- Selenium – 100 mcg
- Magnesium (as Magnesium orotate, or B_{13} magnesium) – 1 g
- Manganese (as Manganese orotate or B_{13} manganese) – 20 mg
- Bromelaine – 600 mg
- Garlic capsules – 6 to 10

High-fibre foods such as pulses, whole grains and all vegetables and fruits are an essential part of the chelation from the body of excess cholesterol.

Following such a programme of chelation as that outlined above calls for a certain dedication, and it is not inexpensive. It is possible to modify the programme and that is what I have suggested in the list of supplements which preceded the discussion of the chelation programme.

One other major method exists by which the self-healing homoeostatic tendencies of the body can be encouraged: fasting, which we will consider in the next chapter.

6
Fasting for Health

Fasting is the oldest method of healing. It is instinctive in sick animals and probably was in primitive humans, too. If carried out sensibly, fasting can also be useful in both treating and preventing disease.

Fasting is often confused with starvation, but strictly speaking it is abstinence for a given time from solid food, but not from liquids.

It is the type of liquids consumed during a fast which has become a somewhat controversial area. Some experts say fasting is effective only if it is undertaken on water only, whereas others, including myself, would advocate that fasting should sometimes be undertaken using fruit and vegetable juices.

Opinion also differs on how long a fast should continue: this largely depends on whether it is being

---

employed to treat ill-health or as a method of preventative medicine, or simply to improve well-being.

For most people a few days of fasting can do nothing but good and can often mean the beginning of recovery from ill-health. It is imperative, however, that no one attempts a long fast unless under the supervision of the experienced practitioner.

Fasting is useful in most cases of physical illness, but there are certain circumstances where it should not be used without qualified supervision. Anyone –

- with an ulcer
- with a history of gout
- who is pregnant
- who has diabetes
- who has heart disease which requires constant medication
- who is regularly taking steroid medication (cortisone, for example)
- who has kidney disease
- who has cancer
- who has an eating disorder of any sort
- who is afraid of the idea of fasting

– should seek professional advice before trying any self-treatment with fasting.

In most of these conditions fasting can be helpful, but needs to be monitored and supervised in case of unusual reactions, especially if there is or has been regular medication.

This warning does not mean that fasting is unsuitable for these conditions, but it does mean that expert help is required to decide on the type of fast, and how long it should be maintained.

There are some strange things that might happen to the body during a fast as toxic debris which has been stored (dumped?) in the fatty tissues is released, and it is best to understand them before beginning so that there is no anxiety when these things happen; they are usually not serious and are often no more than signs of recovery from illness and of detoxification in action.

Symptoms during Fasting

The sort of signs you can expect to notice are:

- a furred tongue
- bad breath
- feeling colder than usual
- feeling 'flu-like' symptoms
- headache and nausea
- production of dark and often offensive urine
- the voiding of amazing accretions from the bowels.

The degree and intensity of these signs of the body cleansing itself of accumulated toxic waste will vary greatly from person to person, often depending on the underlying health and vitality of the individual, as well as the type of fast being used.

Surprisingly, hunger is often not noticed after the first day.

Fasting can be seen as a preparation for spontaneous self-healing by the body. It is not a 'cure' for anything in particular but provides the body with a chance to eliminate toxins which may be preventing the body from functioning normally or from healing itself. So it is important not to treat the initial signs of fasting, such as a 'sick' headache, with any drugs or potions that will suppress them. The headache will go and the tongue will again become pink and healthy again after the fast. All other symptoms will disappear too.

A short fast may not be long enough for all these things to happen, but by repetition the intensity of elimination of the first fast will disappear until, in time, fasts may be enjoyed without marked symptoms and with a noticeable change in health, in terms of energy and clarity of mind.

An area of controversy in fasting is the use of enemas, colonic irrigation and laxatives. There are times when one of these may be called for. If, however, there is no history of constipation, and general health is good, then enemas, etc. are seldom necessary during or after a fast.

If a chronic illness is involved, however, especially of the bowel, or if there exists an allergic or catarrhal condition, then there is a good case for daily enemas or a herbal laxative being given before and after the short fast. There are no rigid rules regarding this, but it is important to recognize that the state of health of the bowel largely determines the degree of health of the body.

Health is impossible without a healthy digestive system, and fasting is one of the best ways of encouraging this.

Supplements During the Fast

Supplements of 'friendly' bacteria (*acidophilus* and *bifidus*) are a definite aid to healthy digestion and internal detoxification. These bacterial cultures are therefore recommended during the fast, but no other supplements should be taken during this period of 'physiological rest'.

During and After the Fast

Breaking the fast correctly is also important. After any length of time without solid food there must be a gentle transition back to full diet.

It is also important that during a fast some gentle exercise is taken; staying in bed is seldom called for, but plenty of rest is necessary. So it is unwise to fast while carrying on normal work.

It is also unwise, and contraindicated, to drive during a fast because dizziness may occur. Fresh air and rest are important, as is the avoidance of stress, which explains the popularity of health farms and hydros, which can offer a restful environment and pleasant diversions such as massage and hydrotherapy during this period of detoxification.

How Often and How Long?

Three-day fasts, undertaken over a weekend, are a good introduction to the experience, and the protocol and details of such an exercise have been set out and described below.

It is necessary to set aside a weekend for such fasting, during which you drop all major obligations and duties. A three-day detoxification every four to six weeks, over six or twelve months, will provide a dramatic improvement in health in most people, and will help to normalize hypertension.

A light meal can be eaten midday on a Saturday, followed by juice on Saturday evening through to Sunday evening, with the fast being broken Sunday evening or Monday morning. This 24- to 36-hour fast every week or fortnight will be extremely beneficial to health.

Alternatively you might prefer to fast for one day each week.

In all cases the aim of a fast is to rest the body from the constant onslaught of food.

The principles involved in fasting can also be applied to everyday eating to make us feel more vital and lively. For instance, breakfast implies that we have been, for a period, without food. This is literally true if the last meal of the previous day was at 6 p.m. and breakfast is at 7 or 8 a.m. But if we eat after 9 at night then the digestive system will barely have finished coping with the evening meal before the next food starts to arrive. Such a pattern of eating helps to make people feel sluggish and lethargic.

By eating earlier in the evening, with no snacks later on, you can be livelier in the morning and have a rested digestive system ready for the next day.

Remember, longer fasts should only be undertaken with the help of a qualified nutritionally-orientated health care practitioner, although a short – 24- to 72-hour – fast is safe to apply without supervision unless contraindicated (see list above).

Preparing for a Fast

The day before: a herbal laxative such as psyllium seeds, a broth made of flax seed (linseed), or castor oil should be taken after the midday meal, which should itself be light (vegetarian for preference, such as a mixed salad or a vegetable soup).

In the evening: have a light fruit meal including pears, apple or grapes, or instead of fruit have a vegetable broth – see recipe below.

Vegetable Broth Recipe

- Use organically grown vegetables if possible. If not, scrub vegetables well before use.
- Into 2.2 litres (4 pints/10 cups) of spring water, place 200 g (4 cups) of finely chopped beetroot, carrots, thick potato peelings, parsley, courgette (zucchini) and leaves of beetroot or parsnip.
- Use no sulphur-rich vegetables such as cabbages or onions, which might produce gas.
- Simmer for five minutes over a low heat to allow for the breakdown of the vegetable fibre and the release of nutrients into the liquid.
- Cool and strain, using only the liquid and not the left-over vegetable content.
- Don't add salt as this broth will contain ample natural minerals which are rapidly absorbed, thus

providing nutrients without straining the digestive system.
- This broth is alkaline and neutralizes any acidity resulting from the fast.
- Drink at least 570 ml (1 pint/2½ cups) of this broth daily during the fast.

On rising the next day: drink either camomile or peppermint tea (unsweetened), or a cup of vegetable broth, or a cup of half spring water and half carrot juice, beetroot juice, or warm or cold apple juice.

A selection of one of these items or bottled spring water should be consumed at two- to three-hourly intervals during the day, making sure that the vegetable broth is consumed at least twice during the day (not less than 570 ml daily) and that the total liquid intake is not less than 2 litres (4 pints), and not more than 4 litres (8 pints) daily.

If fresh vegetable juice is not obtainable, then *Biotta* vegetable juice, available at most health food stores, is suitable for use in fasting as it contains no preservatives (other than lactic acid) and is guaranteed organically grown.

Carrot and beetroot are the ideal juices.

Continue this pattern for the two or three days of the fast.

Finish the fast by eating, on the evening of the final day, one of the following 'meals':

- purée of cooked apple or pear, or
- purée of carrot plus a little puréed vegetable soup, or
- live natural yogurt.

Chew all food very thoroughly and slowly when breaking a fast.

The next morning, eat yogurt and grated apple, or a fresh pear meal, and have a salad and jacket potato for the lunch meal, continuing thereafter on a normal pattern of eating.

The advice for ending a fast depends upon a person not being sensitive to any of the foods mentioned. If dairy produce, for example, is in any way suspect then it should play no part in breaking a fast.

For this reason, anyone with suspected allergies should take advice or be under some degree of supervision during this time.

If necessary a herbal laxative or castor oil could be used on the last evening of the fast, or a warm water enema may be used.

If the individual involved is chronically ill, then daily, small warm water enemas should be used during the fast. The hygiene of the bowel can be further improved by employing one or all of the following during the fast, and for a week or so afterwards:

- Half of a teaspoon of *Lactobacillus acidophilus* and half a teaspoon of *Bifidobacteria* culture daily (good health stores stock freeze-dried cultures of these friendly bacteria). These highly concentrated products will enhance the flora of the bowel.

Note: There are also versions which are suitable for people who are milk sensitive.

If bowel toxicity is a factor (chronic constipation for example):

Stir 1 teaspoon of fine green clay powder (make sure it is a French source – obtainable from many health stores) into a small glass of spring water and allow it to settle, for an hour. Drink the water, but not the sediment. Do this at least once a day during the fast and for a week after. The clay has a detoxi-fying quality and soothes the bowel.

Alternative to Fasting – Monodiets

By definition a monodiet is one in which only a single food is eaten for a period of time. Probably the most famous is the 'grape-cure' which has been used for many years as a means of treating chronic disease. There are a number of variations, however those included in this text relate only to cardiac and hyper-tension problems.

Because this is not a true fast, a monodiet pattern can continue for longer without risk; nevertheless it is suggested that four days is the longest anyone should undertake such a diet without expert supervision and approval.

Note

If a monodiet is to be followed then ensure that the source of the food chosen is organic, unsprayed and free of all chemical preservatives.

- Grapes – especially black ones – are suggested for cardiac conditions, arthritis and blood pressure problems (grapes are rich in potassium). Again, as they will be organically grown (if not then do not start a monodiet) eat the skins (and pips) as well.
- Whole (brown) rice monodiets – recommended for high blood pressure and as an excellent detoxification method.

General Information

A monodiet involves eating just one food of your choice for up to four days (as a rule, if a longer period is needed then just as in fasting, professional advice is needed, and possibly supervision).

On monodiet days drink not less than 1½ litres (3 pints) of water, and not more than 3 litres (6 pints). Drink a little whenever thirsty. Too little water intake may induce constipation.

Quantities of Food on Monodiet Days

On each day of the monodiet, not more than 1.3 kg (3 lb) weight of the selected fruit should be eaten, in small amounts, throughout the day.

A famous American naturopath, Paavo Airola, in describing a grape diet has the patient eat no more than a few grapes at breakfast and lunch on the first day and a few ounces in the evening. On the second day he suggests several ounces at each meal, with a gradual increase in quantity so that by the fourth day as much as is desired is eaten – of grapes only, of course – with an upper limit of 1.3 to 2 kg (3 to 4 lb).

If unprocessed (whole) rice has been selected for a monodiet – and this is specifically known to influence blood pressure beneficially – then 454 g (1 lb) **dry weight (i.e. before cooking)** of an organic source of the food should be the maximum per day. This should be cooked conservatively by placing the washed rice in a saucepan and covering the rice with water. This is brought to the boil and then simmered until soft (all the water having been absorbed). If then allowed to stand for 10 minutes it will be ready to eat. When the rice/grain has cooled it should be divided into servings (five or six servings out of this quantity, since each measure of rice becomes three measures once cooked). When eaten each serving should have added to it a half-dessertspoonful of olive oil and the juice of one lemon (some people add tamari sauce). Cooked rice remains palatable and safe to eat for up to five days if kept in a cool, dry place.

Expect to feel lethargic during a fast or monodiet (less so on the monodiet), and perhaps a little colder than usual, so wear an extra layer of clothing. Rest as much as possible, since the whole object is to allow energy to be employed towards healing and detoxification, not diffused in unnecessary activity.

Take no medication of any sort during a fast without expert approval.

In people of normal weight the fast will result in a number of predictable and beneficial effects, but it won't have the same physiological response in very overweight individuals. For example, growth hormone is released by the pituitary gland during fasting in individuals of normal weight, but this production is reduced in the overweight (growth hormone has many functions, including fat mobilization). Thus, if the fast is undertaken for weight control it must of necessity be a long fast, and it is vital that this be under strict supervision.

A short fast by an overweight person is quite in order, provided their general health is stable and that health enhancement, not weight loss, is the objective.

Fasting is safe if employed correctly, and is one of the swiftest detoxifying and health-promoting methods available.

Try it regularly and you will probably be hooked on it for life, which, if animal studies are any guide, will be longer than if you do not fast regularly.

Blood pressure is certain to drop during a fast, and with repetition as outlined – together with the other measures already discussed – you now have a self-help programme which can give you extra years of healthy life with a stable blood pressure.

Index